MW00938127

The Fearless Smile:
Overcoming Dental Phobia

How to Restore Your Teeth, Youth, and Confidence

The information in this book represents the opinions of the
authors. This information is not intended to treat, diagnose, cure
or prevent any disease. All information provided in this book is
provided for informational purposes only. Information obtained
from this book is not exhaustive and does not cover all diseases,
ailments, physical conditions or their treatment. Each patient's
individual needs are unique. Always seek the advice of your physician, dentist and/or other qualified health care provider with any
questions you have regarding a dental, medical or mental condition before undertaking any procedure, treatment, or health care
regimen set out in this book.

We dedicate this book to the thousands of patients who have had the courage to overcome their dental phobia. Their successful journey has been an inspiration to us and has given us a tremendous amount of professional and personal satisfaction.

All the stories in this book are true—real experiences of patients treated at the authors' private practices in New York City. The names have been changed to protect the privacy of patients.

Table Of Contents

"Sometimes your joy is the source of your smile, but sometimes your smile can be the source of your joy."

— Nhat Hanh

PREFACE

Susan was a woman who seemed to be flourishing in every area. She had a great education, the stable career she'd always dreamed of, a beautiful home, a loving husband, and two wonderful children. To everyone she knew, it really looked like she had a dream life.

But when you would talk to her, you could see that there was still one thing missing. Why didn't Susan ever smile?

Susan's neighbors, colleagues, and even friends blamed it on her smugness and not too pleasant personality. They viewed her as unapproachable and unfriendly. But they did not know the truth—that in fact, she had a deeply hidden fear she couldn't seem to overcome, despite numerous attempts: she was afraid to smile. Back when she was a child, she had a horrible dental experience that traumatized her so much that afterwards she could not force herself to see a dentist again. Over the following years without dental care, her teeth had grown worse and worse, but Susan was still scared to do anything about it. So rather than address the growing problems in her mouth and the unattractive look of her teeth, she simply stopped smiling. It's like somebody who's insecure about her body chooses to wear baggy clothes to hide it. Susan did not know there was a solution within her reach, so she lived with her unhappiness.

Does this story seem familiar to you? Are you overwhelmed with fears and feel that help is nowhere to be found? Not anymore. In this book, you will find real answers. A new smile is within your reach.

Dental Phobia is real, and it affects many people around the globe regardless of their socioeconomic status. Anxiety about dentistry—and avoidance of dental care as a result—negatively influences not just oral health, but also the general, physical, and mental well-being of an individual.

After speaking with so many patients, we have noticed a similar pattern: a history of a traumatic dental experience leads to a culmination of problems that seem insurmountable. We have heard countless times from patients that they didn't know where to turn while the problem was getting out of hand. By writing this book, we wanted to let the millions of people suffering from Dental Phobia to know that help is available.

There is a personal and professional satisfaction that we receive from watching the transformation that patients undergo, once they are able to leave their dental fears behind and have the smile they have always wanted. Once they are free to smile, their health, self-image, self-esteem, and hence their professional and private lives dramatically improve. It's the most rewarding part of our job!

Through initial research on this topic in preparation for this book, we discovered that all phobias share many similarities. It is important to know the psychological roots of any phobia in order to overcome it. The cooperation between a psychologist and a dental specialist seems like a natural and logical union to address all questions and concerns about the complex subject of Dental Phobia.

It is our hope that if you are suffering from dental fear, this book will help you understand -- and ultimately overcome-- your phobia, and step up to a new fearless you with a smile you deserve!

> *"Let us always meet each other with smile, for the smile is the beginning of love."*
> — Mother Teresa

> *"Allowing yourself to smile takes 99% of the effort."*
> — Simon Travaglia

CHAPTER 1

The Basics of Dental Phobia

What Is Dental Phobia?

Dental phobia is a fear or anxiety of going to the dentist that is so extreme, a person worries constantly about or avoids any dental appointment. The distress will actually extend even beyond dental situations, too, so that it is difficult for the person to sleep, perform everyday functions, or even think about anything aside from the fear.

For many patients, enjoying the benefits of a healthy and beautiful smile can seem unattainable—they're too crippled by fear to even imagine visiting a dentist. While people deal with phobias of all kinds of things, dental fear is especially difficult, as it keeps patients from seeking and receiving the dental care they truly need. Psychologists refer to this as *symptoms preventing treatment.*

Dental Fear and Anxiety Affects Health and Confidence

Dentists know firsthand how powerful fear can be. It

prevents patients from taking care of their teeth, leading them to neglect their smiles for years or even decades. It cripples otherwise successful people from moving forward in life. It contributes to problems that keep growing—leading many patients to feel like they wake up one day to enormous dental problems that suddenly feel overwhelming.

The good news is that even when the problems seem insurmountable, there is still hope. The right dentists can provide treatment while still being sensitive to the severe psychological issues associated with oral care. Because dentists who specialize in treating phobic patients deal with this every day, they understand how past negative experiences play into all of these feelings and there is no need to feel awkward or embarrassed about them.

The "Root" of the Problem

Dental sedation experts fully understand the complex relationship between dental fear and neglect. When fear causes a person to avoid going to the dentist, it means missing regular dental checkups and professional hygiene procedures that are essential to taking care of one's teeth. People don't do it on purpose, but because of fear—and that fear drives them to do anything to avoid confronting what they're afraid of. They become anxious and irrational. All that matters is staying away from the bad memories or expected pain of going to the dentist. That is how they unwillingly let the health of their smiles go. Over time, the complications of that neglect will affect a person's oral and mental health, eventually leading to problems with self-esteem and confidence. These patients are not avoiding the dentist, they are avoiding anticipated misery!

The way it usually happens is simple. First, fear will make the patient miss some routine cleanings. Then, a little sensitivity in a tooth arises. Rather than going to the dentist, the person will go to the drugstore and buy a topical numbing solution. This helps the pain go away, even if temporarily, but it often returns, requiring more numbing solution, because the underlying cause of the pain hasn't been addressed. Eventually, the pain becomes intolerable. At that point, most patients end up running to the first oral surgeon that can put them under general anesthesia and take the tooth out while asleep. This goes on for years, one tooth at a time. More teeth are removed, more pain arises, continually snow-balling and changing their smiles. In an effort to avoid pain, they are losing teeth and seeing a negative change in their appearance. They feel unattractive. They are insecure. They lack confidence in increasing areas of life.

Finally, the situation gets to a point where the problems and fear are consuming them. Anxiety over a bad smile consumes people's energies, occupies all their thoughts, and are unable to move on from how they let themselves get to this point. <u>They frankly don't know where to go</u>. They know that their situation is way too advanced for the local general dentist.

Plus, after all the years of neglect and pain, their phobias are stronger than ever. So for most of these patients, even if they find a good dental specialist who is skilled to treat them, they are scared of what treatments they will have to endure to correct past problems. Such patients need more than a good dentist; they need an exceptional dental experience where all their fear, anxiety, and phobias can melt away. This book is about how patients can receive both the skill and the positive experience they need to fix their smile and improve their lives.

Dental fear is a serious matter. But the good news is that there is a solution. Going to the dentist does not need to be a terrifying experience. Thanks to modern technologies and specialists who are committed to improving the process, dental treatment can now be a painless, comfortable, and even enjoyable experience.

Jennifer's Story

One Woman's Journey

As one of the chief officers at a large financial firm, Jennifer regularly had 5,000 people at her disposal to do what she told them to do; yet, the one thing in her life that she couldn't control, that she had never been able to control, was her dental fear.

At first, she was embarrassed to even visit the dentist. It was definitely difficult for her to face her fear, as it is for most fearful patients. They all have that same thing in common: dental anxiety. But in her case, as in so many others, that fear was virtually eliminated through IV sedation.

It took Jennifer a lot of courage to make that initial consultation, but she simply had no choice. Her tooth pain was so intense that she could not sleep, eat, or function well at her job. From her first visit, Jennifer was made to feel comfortable. Her initial consultation was in a cozy room with a comfortable sofa and the relaxing aroma of vanilla scented candles. This was very different from her dreaded fear of having to sit in a dental chair. During her visit, she explained that although she knew that she had many problems with her teeth, she only wanted to focus on the cause of her pain. Her new dentists were understanding and comforting, responded with no lectures about her condition, and promised to give Jennifer a positive experience and a high level of care. Jennifer was also reassured that her smile would always look presentable throughout her treatment. Thanks to the advanced technologies, she could continue her daily routine without people noticing that she was undergoing dental rehabilitation.

The first treatment was to address the cause of her pain. In this case, one of Jennifer's front teeth needed to be removed. During her visit, she was given IV sedation and was safely guided into a state of complete relaxation. Once comfortably sedated, her dental specialists removed the tooth and installed a dental implant. A new temporary tooth was made on the implant which perfectly matched her existing teeth. Jennifer awoke not only to a new tooth, but to a new lease on life. This experience showed her that all the years of neglect and fear could be reversed comfort-

ably and correctly when the skill of highly trained dentists and the experience of IV sedation come together.

Jennifer healed up beautifully from the procedure. She returned for a follow-up visit one week later and reported that she had experienced a pain-free healing. She realized, for the first time in her adult life, that her fear could be conquered. Not long after this, Jennifer decided to treat herself to a smile makeover. All of her dental problems were treated while under IV sedation, and she completed her treatment with a beautiful, healthy smile.

Causes of Dental Phobia

When we probe into the reasons for dental fear, there's oftentimes a history of a bad experience or a negative childhood dental experience. It triggers this fear and anxiety that causes patients to neglect their oral health. Neglect is a slippery slope. It doesn't start out as a big deal, but over the years the effects compound. All of a sudden, patients end up with big dental issues and start losing teeth altogether and it wreaks havoc on their lives.

Just like a person with acrophobia feels terrified of heights or someone with agoraphobia hates being in public places, someone with dental phobia fears the dentist. Phobias come from all kinds of sources, whether real or imagined. It might be because of childhood issues, because of previous bad experiences, or from no obvious cause at all; whatever the case, phobias usually send patients into panic and fear, increasing their heart rates, shortening their breath, and making them tremble. Phobias cripple people from being able to function normally and, in the case of dental fear, can cause serious health-related consequences.

Why People Are Afraid of the Dentist

The statistics regarding dental phobias make one thing pretty clear: dental phobia is a very common problem, across all ages, personalities, and vocations. There are so many different levels of fear and so many different people affected by it. Some patients may feel just a little uneasy; some worry for a few days ahead of an appointment; still others are absolutely terrified. While not everyone needs sedation, virtually everyone feels some sense of nervousness. Truthfully, even dentists can get a little apprehensive when undergoing treatment— some degree of fear is normal and common.

Fear of the Unknown

There are many reasons people are afraid of dentists. Mostly, it's the fear of the unknown—the same root that's behind most phobias. People wonder what treatment will feel like and if anything will hurt; but mostly, they just don't know what to expect. And not knowing what to expect often leads to preparation for the worst. From sudden, sharp pains in the middle of a procedure to not feeling numb enough, to enormous needles ready to generate terrible pain.

Invasion of Privacy

Dentists work in a very private part of the body that also happens to be home to many nerve endings. The mouth is sensitive to two of the body's five major senses, taste and touch. While this is good for culinary purposes, it can make dental treatment more frightening, as even the smallest touch is magnified in perception.

The sensory information produced by the slightest touch from a dentist can be transmitted to the brain as a major sensation. And because we are not used to touches inside our mouth other than feeling food, teeth, and maybe a kiss, the feeling is foreign and often not pleasant. Even though the tools dentists use are generally quite small, because they are foreign to the receptors in the mouth, they may feel very large. Any manipulation a dentist makes of the oral cavity feels awkward, uncomfortable, and much more intense than it would in other places on the body. Our mouths are suited for the sense of taste. That is what they are for. Our skin, on the other hand, is better suited for the sense of touch and reacts more appropriately to touch. The work dentists perform would be much more tolerable if it weren't taking place in the mouth.

Invasion of Personal Space

Receiving dental care is also a major invasion of personal space. Generally, people stay an arm's length apart. Even spouses respect personal space. But for dentists to care for your smile, it requires them to get uncomfortably close, right into the midst of your mouth, which is a very private and personal body part.

Negative Childhood Experiences

Another cause of dental phobia is very negative childhood dental experiences. Most dentists would attest to the fact that a high percentage of dental fear or anxiety links directly to this same root. What's more, this connection has been confirmed by research: in fact, one study showed that as many as 85% of dental fears stem from childhood experiences.

For one thing, previous generations grew up in times when dental technology was very far behind what is available today. No matter how many times we hear the anecdotes, it's still shocking when patients tell dental horror stories. These patients say, "Do you believe when I was a child they didn't even have Novocain? There was no numbing."

Others will remember going to the dentist as horribly painful and will say things like, "My dentist was a butcher."

As one powerful example, there were dental offices all over the world years ago that didn't use any local anesthesia (novocain) for children. Those kids have grown up into middle-aged adults, scarred for life by those horrible memories. Many have avoided dental visits completely as a result of what happened when they were children. It's terrible what these memories can do to kids. It gives them preconceived negative notions of what to expect at the dentist.

Television, especially kids' cartoons, is also notorious for portraying dentists as being scary to go to. For example, *Finding Nemo,* a popular children's movie, has a character that is a dentist and he is portrayed as terribly frightening: a crazy man who yields large, loud, scary tools. Television shapes the view our society has of dentists being villains.

Parents may also be responsible for their children's dental phobias. Research shows that there's a major connection between parental and child dental fear, especially in kids eight years old and younger.

Mothers and Fathers tell their children, "Oh, you're going to the dentist today. It's going to hurt! They're going to use a long needle." Some parents unfortunately use the threat of going to the dentist as a punishment, saying things like, "You better be good, because if you don't behave, I'm going to take you right to the dentist!"

Rhoda's Story:

A Bad Experience as a Child Can Last a Lifetime

Dental phobias oftentimes begin in childhood. Take Rhoda, a happily married middle-aged businesswoman and mother of two. In most of her life, she's the vision of success: just promoted at work, owns a beautiful house in the suburbs, is actively involved in her kids' soccer games, even makes time to volunteer in her community. Yet in one area of her life, she's utterly powerless and filled with anxiety: she is terrified of going to the dentist.

According to Rhoda, it all started in elementary school

when her parents would tease her about going to the dentist as a form of punishment: "If you get in trouble again, we're gonna take you to the dentist!" and "Don't worry, the needle will only hurt a little bit." Then, when she did have to go, the experience was rushed and uncomfortable: she still remembers the gruff voice of the dentist and the unmistakable dental office smell. As a result, she stopped going as soon as she could, and her teeth suffered the consequences: severe decay, gum disease, crowns, root canals, and major pain. Today she wishes she could have overcome that fear to save herself all the heartache later.

On the flip side, concerned parents can totally change the dental experience for their kids in a positive way, helping them to avoid dental phobias later in life.

Here are two things parents should do:

1. **Be supportive!** Think of the way you talk about going to the dentist. Avoid joking about it being painful or scary. It should be a fun place that your child enjoys visiting. Set the stage for it to be that way by the words and tone you use to describe it.

2. **Find a dentist that caters to kids!** Pediatric dentists specialize in making dentistry child-friendly with colorful offices, trained staff, and cute nicknames like "sleepy juice" for Novocain and "Mr. Thirsty" for the suction.

CHAPTER 2

Understanding Phobias

In order to fully understand the dynamics of dental fear, it is important to know the basic characteristics of fear and anxiety in general terms. All phobias, fears, and anxieties have a unifying commonality and pattern.

What Is an Anxiety?

An anxiety is a difficult uneasiness in the mind, usually relating to an impending or anticipated event that is perceived as negative.

What Is a Phobia?

A phobia is a persistent, irrational fear of a specific object, activity, or situation that leads to a compelling desire to avoid it.

Veronica's Story

How Phobia Nearly Ruined a Career

Veronica had an excellent record as a trial lawyer. She was considered to be both a quick thinker on her feet as well as a clever courtroom tactician. When she won twice in appellate court, she quickly attained celebrity status within the firm. Nonetheless, she had been passed over for partner because she refused airline travel and thus was not able to visit the firm's corporate clients on the West Coast.

Veronica wanted to advance her career so badly that she decided to take things into her own hands. Instead of going in for treatment for her phobia or starting slowly with a short flight, she impulsively flew to California to visit one of the firm's important clients who had complained of her "unwillingness" to fly. After about an hour into the cross-country flight, she began to emotionally unravel. She became increasingly agitated and couldn't stop fixating on two overweight women in front of her, both seated on the right side of the plane's cabin. Drained of any remaining self-control, she stood up and screamed, "You girls are really fat! I want one of you to get off your fat butt and sit on the other side of the aisle so the plane is balanced and won't tip over." Naturally, they refused.

In her state of panic, she ran towards the door of the plane yelling that she was going to jump out. Although it is impossible for the door of an airborne commercial jet to be opened from the inside by a passenger, Veronica was tackled and restrained by several passengers and flight attendants. At this point, she was fully hysterical. Unable to keep her under control they put her in a strait jacket. One of the worst things possible for a person in her condition! When she wouldn't stop screaming, they gagged her.

When they finally landed in California, federal marshals came on the plane and led her away in handcuffs. Several days later, she took a train back to New York and, after finally admitting to herself that she had a problem she could not fix by herself, she began treatment for fear of flying. The clinical psychologist who treated her diagnosed her with extreme aviophobia (fear of flying) in combination with claustrophobia (fear of being in closed places).

After identifying Veronica's problem, her therapist was able to come up with a treatment plan, combining biofeedback with virtual reality therapy. She learned how to breathe in a way that would lead to relaxation (slow abdominal breathing) and could practice in a safe environment (a virtual airplane) before embarking on an actual airline flight. When she was ready to fly, her doctor encouraged her to take it slowly and begin with a short trip from New York City to Syracuse, eventually building up to longer flights. Now, Veronica is flying all over the country to meet with her clients. She was finally named partner at her law firm and was able to take a celebratory and long-awaited vacation in Europe.

Phobias are irrational fears about objects, people or situations. Phobias, along with obsessive compulsive disorders and addictions, have a tendency to be progressive in nature. Therefore, if left untreated, they usually worsen over time. There is no rhyme or reason as to how and why phobias develop and there is rarely, if ever, a single identifiable cause. Almost everyone experiences occasional bouts of anxiety in the absence of a realistic threat, but what makes phobic behavior distinct is that irrational fears and concerns begin to govern important decisions, eventually becoming disruptive to the lives of the individual and those close to him. In retrospect, many phobic patients can recall this point of disruption, often referring to it as a time when they "crossed over"; a point in which the phobia begins to dominate a person's thoughts and behaviors, taking on almost obsessional characteristics.

Phobias have absolutely nothing to do with intelligence. They are not about reasoning or facts, but are a physical reaction to anxiety. One aspect of phobia that leads to a great deal of frustration is that while a phobic person is usually aware that their fear is unreasonable, it is impossible for them to overcome the fear or confront the situation in a reasonable manner. For this reason, telling them that there is nothing to be afraid of will only be detrimental to their condition and probably leave the person feeling even more alienated and misunderstood.

As an example, almost all people who have a fear of flying have heard the same statistic: the automobile ride to the airport is far more dangerous than the flight. Because phobias are not related to intelligence or rational understanding, this sort of reasoning is useless and often insulting.

Similarly, reminding a person who has avoided the dentist for a decade that not going for regular cleanings every six months will result in poor dental hygiene and tooth decay will not be helpful advice. The phobic patient certainly knows this and only wishes he were capable of sticking to such a regimen. The problem with phobic behavior is that the ability to think and reason rationally dissolves once the individual is faced with the feared situation and is instantly replaced by dread or raw panic.

Despite this intense feeling of dread and panic, most people never seek help for their debilitating fears. Frequently, people will put off getting help for numerous reasons, which are usually as unrealistic and exaggerated as the phobia itself.

This avoidance is often due to embarrassment or concern that they will be ridiculed. The person may have difficulty admitting their own weakness and feel more comfortable trying to overcome the phobia on their own. This is referred to as "symptoms preventing treatment." People generally have psychological "blind spots" when it comes to seeing themselves objectively, honestly or as others see them.

Phobias typically worsen over time when people behave protectively. This can result in an inability to lead a normal existence and eventually progress to where unrealistic fears control a person's feelings, thoughts and behaviors. For instance, a fear of elevators may prevent a person from taking a job; a fear of having a panic attack on the street may prevent a person from leaving their home; and a fear of the dentist often leads to a patient avoiding the dentist altogether, resulting in mounting dental problems that could become painful, embarrassing and unhealthy.

Fight or Flight

Phobias are actually the body's physical reaction to irrationally perceived danger. The body's normal reaction to danger is known as the "fight or flight" response and is directly linked to self-preservation. When this response is activated you have two options: either stay put and face the lurking danger, or run away in order to avoid confronting the feared situation.

When the body senses fear, muscles naturally tighten and function almost like a suit of armor in an effort to protect vital organs. Blood pressure, respiration and heart rate soar, quickly delivering oxygenated blood to the body's large muscles. Blood flow is temporarily shunted away from the peripheral areas (hands, feet and face) and circulates where it is needed (heart, lungs and other vital organs). This is why when a person is afraid, their hands and feet often become cold and the face can become pale. Hence the statements, "cold hands warm heart," "you look like you've seen a ghost" and "I have cold feet" really do make sense biologically.

The body's physical response to fear dates back to prehistoric times when survival was linked directly to a person's ability to protect himself from the dangers posed by the environment. In early civilizations, the person who was able to react quickly to cues that a saber tooth tiger was in proximity was certainly more likely to survive than the person who snoozed even slightly. This is the basis for Darwin's theory of natural selection or "survival of the fittest" and explains many of the traits that have been carried forward to modern-day man. Concerns about the consequences of not making a mortgage payment may trigger the same warning system as those worries that our ancestors had about becoming prey to saber tooth tigers during prehistoric times. While environmental and emotional concerns have changed throughout history, our tightly wound autonomic nervous systems have always responded to perceived threats in pretty much the same way.

It is only over the past 400-500 years that people living in North America could generally sit around in a relaxed way without any major environmental threat. Given that human beings have walked the earth for hundreds of thousands of years, it is not surprising that we have inherited the instincts of our most alert and vigilant ancestors. Ironically, what kept our ancestors alive has evolved beyond usefulness, and now presents disadvantages.

When a person senses some sort of threat, he not only becomes emotionally aware of impending danger (anxiety), but his body becomes prepared as well. Although in prehistoric times this almost always worked in man's favor, such an extreme reaction to modern-day fears is not always beneficial. Frequent bouts of increased respiration, blood pressure and heart rate put undue strain on the body's systems which may result in serious health problems. This can also lead to protective behavior and, ultimately, avoidance. If you live in a city and every time you hear a loud noise your "fight or flight" response is activated, you will certainly waste vital resources by adopting a defensive psychological posture or mindset. Being thin-skinned or having a short fuse is not a relaxing way to live a life.

Fortunately, strategies have been developed to manage stress and anxiety. While it is natural to be afraid, it is possible to change the way we react to things in our environment that may scare us, but do not present actual threats.

CHAPTER 3

Acupuncture, Relaxation Training and Hypnosis

Acupuncture

Research has shown that acupuncture prior to dental treatment can have a beneficial effect on patient anxiety. In one study observing eight dentists and 20 very anxious patients, there was a significant reduction in fear after undergoing acupuncture treatment: where only six could handle treatment without it, all 20 were able to undergo dental work with it. Additionally, acupuncture has been shown to help patients manage the gagging reflex, a response commonly associated with putting foreign bodies in the mouth. According to one study, a large number of gagging patients can undergo dental work after stimulation of the P-6 Neikuan acupuncture point, located on the wrist.

Relaxation Training

Relaxation training, also known as progressive muscle relaxation, systematic muscle relaxation, or Jacobson relaxation, is a therapy designed to reduce anxiety and fear through certain techniques that relax muscles. A patient goes into a quiet room and tenses a group of muscles, then relaxes those muscles, and after that does the same with another group of muscles. Throughout the process, he or she focuses on the difference between tense and relaxed muscles. This treatment may also involve meditation, breathing exercises, or yoga. One study reviewing ten years of relaxation training showed consistent, significant improvement of patient anxiety through this treatment.

Hypnosis

The long history of hypnosis attests to its power in behavior modification, particularly in the realm of fear. Research on using hypnosis to treat dental fear shows that it can be helpful when combined with other techniques like systematic desensitization, but it is highly dependent on the individual. With all of these treatment options available, however, it is still difficult to guarantee success. Estimations on the risk of failure are as high as 60% — with a variety of different factors to blame, including insufficient motivation, fear bigger than the treatment, accidents during treatment, and others. What today's dental patients need is a stronger treatment option, one that can address all levels of fear.

CHAPTER 4

Psychotherapy

The Role of Psychotherapy in Treating Phobias

When patients first come for treatment, it is not un-common for them to be frightened to even talk about their phobia. Their phobia has usually been an ex-tremely stressful and often embarrassing aspect of their lives, which may be a source of deep shame. There is often a fear of being seen as weak, ignorant or com-pletely crazy. Although we cannot know for sure why certain people become phobic about particular things, it is likely that genetics contribute to the tendency to exhibit phobic behavior. Many patients find it a relief to hear that it is not their fault and has nothing to do with character or intelligence, but is simply a neurological "glitch" and can be corrected through a combination of behavioral therapies.

Cognitive Therapy

Teaching Rational Thinking

Cognitive therapy teaches the patient to become aware of the connection between their thoughts and moods. This is achieved by assigning written homework in which the patient monitors negative thoughts that are typically exaggerated. Patients are taught to substitute these thoughts with more reality based ideas. Once the patient has an understanding of the thoughts fueling their fears, they are encouraged to complete tasks that involve confronting their fears and reacting in the ways they have been taught. In order to ease into the treatment, they start with low-demand tasks and work up to more difficult ones.

For example, consider a person who is very fearful of public speaking. Almost always, underlying such a fear is the irrational belief that it will be catastrophic if they do not perform well. Teaching the person to think more rationally in the situation will result in lessening the feeling of anxiety. The goal is learning to replace catastrophic thinking with more reasonable or rational thinking. Therapy is not completed until the patient exhibits the ability to change in the therapist's office as well as in the real world under actual stress, a process called generalization.

Behavioral Therapy

Teaching People to Smile

The basis for behavioral therapy is that when you change the way people behave, emotions and corresponding beliefs will follow, not just the other way around. "Laughter yoga", in which people meet in groups for the sole purpose of laughing to feel good, supports this theory.

Additionally, research done by Fritz Strack, a psychologist at the University of Wurzburg in Germany, shows that mimicking emotional expression triggers a matching emotional response. In Strack's study, using a "pen-in mouth procedure," he found that people felt happier and responded more positively to stimuli such as cartoons when they held a pen between their teeth, allowing them to smile, than when they held it between their lips, forcing a frown.

People with poor dental health tend to smile and laugh far less frequently than people who are happy with their teeth. This is an added incentive to the patients hoping to overcome their dental phobia. In addition to renewed dental health, an improved emotional state is also a likely outcome.

Cognitive Behavioral Therapy (CBT) for treating phobias includes tools for relaxation training as well as gradual desensitization to the feared object or situation. Through repeated exposure to the feared object or situation paired with relaxation training, desensitization teaches the patient to react in a positive way rather than retreating into a state of panic. This is also referred to as "building in a competing response." As a result of genetics and experience, individuals respond in predictable ways to certain external factors or life events. The behavioral therapist's job is to reteach the patient and change the way they react to certain stimuli, resulting in positive and long-lasting change. Although making these changes can seem extremely difficult and uncomfortable, learning to challenge long-held but never tested belief systems has proven extremely effective over the long-term.

For instance, the criminal continues a life of crime because the violent acts give him some sort of a rush or high. If the same criminal is forced to feel sick or have an unappealing sensation while he is involved in criminal activity he will eventually cease this type of behavior. This example of classical conditioning was brought to life in the 1962 novella by Anthony Burgess, *A Clockwork Orange*. The important difference is that present-day behavioral therapists use positive reinforcement to encourage people to change their behavior. Punishment and negative reinforcement are never used.

Cognitive Behavioral Therapy (CBT)

The Combined Effects

As the name implies, CBT uses a combination of both cognitive and behavioral techniques. Cognitive therapy focuses on the idea that people can be taught to think in more effective ways, while behavioral therapy works under the premise that human behaviors are learned and therefore can be unlearned. In combination, these techniques can provide the phobic patient with powerful tools for reducing anxiety and successfully conquering fears. The approach not only provides a means of changing the ways people view themselves and their environment (cognitions), but also the ways in which they act in that environment (behaviors).

As opposed to other therapies, CBT techniques are known to generate results that are both durable and quick. On average, effective CBT therapy takes six months to a year, while other more traditional forms of therapy, like psychodynamic psychotherapy and psychoanalysis, can take years, and even decades. The harder-working patient will see results more quickly, especially if he practices what is learned during sessions outside of the office. When a patient starts therapy, it is made clear that, at some point, together the therapist and client will have to make the decision to end treatment. Therefore, CBT is not an open-ended, never-ending process. Patients are often surprised to hear their CBT therapist hinting at termination issues, something many patients say they never heard before from a therapist.

CBT is extremely effective in treating phobias and anxiety through systematic desensitization or exposure therapy, providing tools to reduce anxiety and encourage relaxation when coming into contact with a phobic situation. CBT involves gradual encounters, first in the imagination or in a virtual environment and then in reality. The patient eventually realizes that while the situation may be unpleasant, it is not harmful. With each exposure, there is an increased sense of control over the phobia. It is so effective because, in reality, our *thoughts* control our feelings and behaviors, not external things, like people, situations, and events (the things we fear).

CBT also provides the phobic patient with tools for relaxation which are very helpful in managing stress. A combination of biofeedback and virtual reality therapy is the most effective method for treating phobias. Virtual reality therapy exposes a person to the phobia in a controlled environment. Biofeedback allows people to see how they are physiologically responding to stress by monitoring heart rate, blood pressure, muscle tension, blood flow, and even brainwaves. In treating phobias, virtual reality alone has a high success rate; but when combined with biofeedback, the success rate increases significantly.

In order for CBT to be effective, exposure is necessary, and the initial exposure should be minimal. Only through systematic, gradually increasing exposures without "running away" or "behaving protectively" will treatment be successful. This is also referred to as graded flooding. *Sedation Dentistry* counters this hurdle by providing a pleasant experience from the start. The patient will automatically become less anxious with each subsequent visit. If a person is so frightened that even sedation dentistry (certainly the most relaxing and painless dental experience possible) is too scary, then the utilization of virtual reality and biofeedback provide an ideal alternative.

Biofeedback

Biofeedback works by teaching the patient to become aware of certain physiological changes in their body. The patient is hooked up to a monitor by placing surface electrodes on the fingertips, abdominal areas, forehead or skull; precisely where the electrodes are placed is determined by the specific type of biofeedback employed. Computerized signals are transferred to a monitor that can read variations in autonomic arousal (e.g., blood pressure, heart rate, and skin temperature).

Biofeedback is used in a variety of ways by CBT therapists. EEG biofeedback (also known as neurofeedback) uses computerized electronic measurement devices that are placed on the surface of the patient's head in order to monitor brainwave activity. This type of biofeedback is very effective in treating patients with ADD/ADHD, anxiety, insomnia, depression, and OCD. When used in treating ADD/ADHD, the computer "feeds back" important information relevant to concentration. Through guided experience the patient is able to learn to significantly increase brainwaves compatible with focus and attention. Ultimately, the patient learns to create "better" brainwaves automatically. Video games (Mattel Inc.) exist to facilitate this process, specifically designed for children with ADD and ADHD. The child will only do well in the game when the "good" kind of brainwaves (beta waves) are activated, therefore making it possible to learn to increase healthy brainwave activity simply by playing a video game.

Neurofeedback can also be used to teach athletes to concentrate better and, therefore, perform better under stress. Golfers who complain they "choke" or get the yips when they putt are often successfully treated with brainwave biofeedback. Canada's 2010 Winter Olympics team's top secret initiative "OWN THE PODIUM" used biofeedback very successfully. The high-tech training gave their athletes a decided edge in their ability to switch rapidly between a relaxed state and a super-focused state, while minimizing the use of valuable physiological resources. The biofeedback equipment used in many CBT offices is the same as that utilized by many professional sports clubs as well as by NASA to prepare astronauts for space exploration (www.thoughttechnology.com).

Biofeedback has also been able to successfully treat tension, or more specifically, tension headaches. Several sensors are attached to the forehead so that tension in the muscles of the head, jaw, and neck can be recorded through these electrodes. Muscular tension is then converted to a tone and any increase in muscular tension leads to an increase in the tone. Consequently, as tension decreases, the tone goes down. The patient is instructed to reduce the tone in ways that correspond to the reduction of tension in that area. After a short period of time, through trial and error, the patient learns how to relax the muscles of the jaw, forehead and neck, thereby reducing symptoms of tension headache. The patient is slowly weaned from the biofeedback machine as he learns to rely on internal signals of relaxation rather than the signals from the machine.

Respiratory Sinus Arrhythmia biofeedback (RSA bio-feedback) is frequently used for the treatment of phobias. By taking measures of change in heart rate and respiration patterns, the patient learns how to breathe more effectively in order to reduce anxiety. Because stress is measured by increases in heart rate and respiration pattern, learning how to effectively control these bodily responses makes it possible to reduce stress in previously anxiety-producing experiences. When slow abdominal breathing (at a rate of 5-7 breaths per minute) is accompanied by rapid increases of heart rate during inhalation and rapid drops in heart rate during exhalation, a state of RSA can be achieved in which it is physiologically impossible to experience anxiety of any kind. In order to achieve this state, the clinical goal is to determine the precise breathing rate that generates the largest swing in heart rate during peak inhalation and exhalation.

Biofeedback makes this possible by combining EKG (or heart rate monitoring), with respiration pattern measures. As in any other type of biofeedback, once the patient has practiced RSA breathing for a period of time with the biofeedback machine, they will become prepared to use it in real-life situations. As explained later, RSA biofeedback combined with Virtual Reality Therapy is an extremely strong tool in combating phobias with a 90% cure rate. There has been a surge of creativity by electrical engineers and neuroscientists that has resulted in technology available to mental health professionals and the general public. It is unfortunate that most people are not aware of this availability, particularly in comparison to the level of exposure that pharmacological products receive. Interested readers are referred to www.bio-medical.com.

Experience reveals that people often need far more than one simple contact to begin the process necessary to make significant behavioral changes. There are various stages of change that encourage people to take these necessary steps that recent advances in technology are now addressing. Fortunately, with advances in the powers of technology customized multi part messaging can now target groups of patients struggling with paralyzing anxiety to exposure leading to increased opportunities to regain control of their lives. Interested readers wanting to learn about these applications are referred to www.digipowers.com.

Virtual Reality Therapy

Virtual Reality Therapy (VRT) immerses the patient into a virtual environment using a head mounted display with a 3-D image, similar to those used for virtual reality games. It creates a visual, auditory, and sensory environment that psychologically exposes the patient to the feared object or activity (e.g., flying in an airplane or speaking in front of a large group of people).

The therapist maintains control of the entire experience, thereby allowing exposure to the portions of the experience that create the most anxiety. Virtual reality programs (at www.virtuallybetter.com) exist for a wide range of phobias and the popularity of this type of therapy continues to grow due to its high success rate when used in combination with biofeedback. Mental health professionals who offer these specialized treatment protocols, considered the gold standard in anxiety management, are required to obtain years of additional training, following their doctoral studies.

Treating Phobias through Biofeedback and VRT

In order to provide maximum effectiveness for phobic patients, the VRT experience is typically paired with a tool for inducing relaxation. This is known as cognitive restructuring. The idea is that if a person can change their psychological state during the virtual experience, with practice, they can be taught to make the same change in real life. Because biofeedback monitors measure physiological reactions to stress, the therapist uses these monitors to make patients aware of their reactions and ultimately teach them how to control these physiological responses.

When a person gets anxious, one of the first reactions is an increased rate of breathing. Instead of breathing from deep down in the diaphragm (also known as abdominal, diaphragmatic or belly breathing), anxious people get caught up in shallow chest breathing (thoracic breathing). Thoracic breathing actually leads to a change in the ratio of oxygen and carbon dioxide, which can result in hyperventilation. When a person hyperventilates, he ends up expelling too much carbon dioxide. This has the unfortunate effect of reducing the efficiency of hemoglobin and its ability to release oxygen as blood travels through the body.

The result is not enough oxygen in the bloodstream and the feeling that you aren't getting enough air. The trouble begins to accelerate as this feeling often leads to panic and inevitably more rapid, shallow chest breathing and increased hyperventilation. This is why people who are panicking are often advised to breath into a paper bag; this forces carbon dioxide back into the lungs. In many cases, this type of reaction can lead to crippling panic attacks. Many emergency room visits are a result of people who believe they are having a heart attack when in reality they are having a panic attack. The symptoms they are experiencing (shortness of breath accompanied by the feeling of suffocation), are remarkably similar to the symptoms of a heart attack.

At the other end of the spectrum, RSA breathing, as explained earlier, temporarily shuts off the body's ability to generate anxiety of any kind. RSA biofeedback has proven to be an essential component of virtual reality treatment. Pairing an individual's specific maximum relaxation RSA rate with the visceral experience associated with the phobia (e.g., flying in virtual reality) represents the "CURE POINT." This makes it possible for relaxation to be associated with an experience that was once only associated with terror. Cognitively, the person starts to actually believe that anticipatory anxiety will no longer be an issue, which ultimately leads to relief of phobic avoidance behavior.

Biofeedback is very effective in teaching the benefits of abdominal breathing, because it gives people a true understanding of how their body responds to the way in which they breathe (whether it makes them more relaxed or more nervous). Without this tool, patients would have no way of knowing precisely when they have achieved the correct cardiac response. Once they have learned the correct breathing pattern they will be able to practice it in conjunction with the virtual reality experience, then without the biofeedback monitor and, eventually, to control anxiety in real-life situations.

Before VRT existed, patients were asked to create images in their mind in order to replicate the feared experience. This was a huge obstacle in the treatment of phobias because it is unrealistic to expect a person to develop realistic imagery about a situation they have typically spent their life avoiding. The use of imagery to combat phobias was an intervention developed in the

1960s by Dr. Joseph Wolpe.

Dr. Wolpe also proposed that the patient's anxiety be measured by having the patient simply rate the level of anxiety he was experiencing on a ten point scale. Technology, in the form of biofeedback monitoring, has fortunately replaced these subjective measures. Dr. Wolpe's treatment protocol represented some great ideas that were only able to become truly effective some forty years later, with the advent of biofeedback and VRT. These emerging technologies have provided a means for Wolpe's theory to become the backbone for a truly effective treatment of phobias, which has provided life-changing results for many phobic patients.

Dawn's Story

Depression & IV Sedation Dentistry

Dawn was diagnosed with clinical depression when she was a teenager and experienced periodic bouts of depression ever since. Some of these bouts lasted longer than others and at times she felt glimpses of relief (even what she thought might be happiness); but for the most part, her thoughts and moods were dominated by gloom and loneliness. She had been on various anti-depressants, but she didn't feel that any of them came close to actually lifting her depression. She had a job she disliked and although she dated, she had never been in a serious long-term relationship.

From the time she graduated from college and was "on her own," she hadn't taken the greatest care of herself. One of the things she neglected was her teeth. She couldn't be bothered with cleanings, especially when she was feeling depressed. One of her worst bouts of depression lasted about two years. After that, she just stopped going to the dentist. She felt embarrassed about her teeth and tried to conceal them whenever possible.

She saw herself as unattractive and was sure she had bad breath. Even though men continued to ask her out, she started saying "no" every time because she couldn't imagine how anyone would really like her, let alone want to kiss her. Caught in the age old cycle that signals low self-esteem, she reasoned that any man without the good sense to steer clear of her must have had such poor judgment that she'd better steer clear of

56

him. Dawn stopped smiling. As her depression worsened, so did her teeth.

Eventually, she was so down in the dumps that she had two options: either do something about it or cease living altogether. One morning, she woke up feeling so bad she thought that it "literally hurt to be" and recognized it was finally time to get help. After a few visits with a therapist who specializes in Cognitive Behavioral Therapy (CBT), a treatment plan was recommended. The psychologist's plan included a behavioral intervention designed to improve her self-esteem. Initial interventions included cognitive rehearsal, use of videotape feedback in CBT oriented group therapy, neurofeedback, cognitive restructuring, aerobic exercise, and stress inoculation training.

When he mentioned to her that her smile seemed to generate excess muscle tension and appeared hidden, Dawn disclosed her ongoing struggle with dental phobia. Like many women of her generation, her first dentist did not use much Novocain and she had been traumatized. Her therapist thought it was important for her to start taking care of her teeth, and because conventional dentistry was out of the question, he suggested sedation dentistry. Her first reaction was that he couldn't possibly understand her if he believed that she could simply start going to the dentist upon his suggestion.

Fortunately, her therapist had anticipated the source of her anxiety and explained why this visit to the dentist would be different from anything she had experienced in the past. She eventually trusted her psychologist enough to schedule an appointment with her new dentist. Initially she was very scared, but thanks to IV sedation, her first treatment visit was pain free and uneventful; she was shocked when she was told she had been in the chair for more than three hours. She was even more surprised to learn that all of her dental work was complete.

Unlike her psychotherapy, which she knew would take at least six months, her dental problems were basically resolved in one day. Although the dental work was completed, it took some time before she was convinced that she didn't have to hide her teeth all the time. Eventually, she started smiling again. Her newfound smile and laughter provided its own therapy. Just as she had learned to avoid the dentist because of her building anxiety, she learned to relax because sedation dentistry turned out to be completely pain free. She remembers thinking to herself, "I wouldn't have believed it if it weren't me; one day I had a phobia and the next day I didn't."

She started taking yoga classes where she found out about laughter yoga*. Her therapist convinced her it was a great idea for her to join a "laughter club." Not because she was especially funny or wanted to become a comedian, but because her CBT therapist knew it would help with her depression. Behave a certain way and your emotions will follow.

*Laughter yoga was started in 1995 by Dr. Madan Kataria (www.laughteryoga.org) popularly known as the Guru of Giggling (London Times). Today there are over 5,000 "laughter clubs" or laughter yoga groups around the world. Laughter is known to have health benefits (both physiological and psychological). Clinical research reveals that the body doesn't distinguish between "fake laughter" and "genuine laughter" and derives similar benefits from both. It is known to relieve stress, boost the immune system, alleviate pain and promote overall health. The benefits of laughter are yet another reason to take care of your smile.

CHAPTER 5

Sedation Dentistry

If every thought you have about a dental examination generates anxiety, the problem can be easily solved: avoid going altogether. Because thoughts of the dentist are associated with anxiety, dismissing these thoughts serves as reinforcement, thereby setting the stage for the phobia to gather steam. Throughout this process, avoiding the dentist altogether, becomes the status quo because the relief that is linked to the avoidance serves as the primary reinforcement. This brings to mind the old saying, "I like to hit myself on the head with a hammer because it feels so good to stop."

Visiting a regular dentist, rather than one specializing in sedation dentistry, will probably serve to justify all of the protective behaviors that support the phobia. The phobic person will most likely become terrified and revert back to their original state. Sedation dentistry conforms to the same basic principles that serve as the backbone of virtual reality/biofeedback therapy. The patient is made to feel at ease and physically comfortable, automatically resulting in the dental experience being linked with "good" feelings. An added benefit is that the patient knows that the majority of their dental problems will be behind them following the first visit. This means a great deal to the person who had terrifying visions of hours upon painful hours in the dentist's chair, drawn out over countless visits.

With dental phobias in particular, it is important for people to find a way to manage their fears. In a recent study of over 6,000 patients in Australia, 29.2% of people with fear had delayed treatment, whereas just 11.6% without fear had done so.

This demonstrates an important reality: without a way to successfully treat that anxiety, it is very likely that a dental patient will delay treatment and exacerbate their oral problems.

Sandy's Story

Finding the Right Dentist
Without Lectures or Judgment

Sandy grew up very afraid to go to the dentist. Her mother also had a fear of the dentist and Sandy still remembers sensing her mother's anxiety. Because her mother was so fearful, she always remained in the waiting room or went out for a walk while Sandy was in the chair. Sandy was sure her dentist left her in the chair for long stretches of time and often felt like he had forgotten about her. She remembered the feeling of fluoride leaking into her throat making her feel like she was going to choke and nobody would be around to help her. She had many cavities as a child and always dreaded going to the dentist. She would always know the date of her next appointment and ruminated about it for weeks. When she ended up going, the expe-

rience was always frightening and painful.

As an adult, Sandy avoided going to the dentist unless she had a toothache that was so painful the tooth had to be removed. As the years went on, her dental health got worse and worse. When she would finally go to the dentist, she had several experiences that were very embarrassing and uncomfortable for her. She recalls a hygienist scolding her repeatedly for not getting enough cleanings and "not taking good enough care of your teeth!" After this humiliating experience she stopped going to the dentist altogether. In addition to inheriting her mother's fear of the dentist, the fact that Sandy never had a nurturing or understanding dentist certainly didn't help matters. Sandy's dental problems continued to escalate. Fortunately, a close friend of hers knew about sedation dentistry and told Sandy about it.

Her friend helped her get to and from her first appointment convincing her that she would be made to feel comfortable at the dentist's office and certainly would not be reprimanded for not taking care of her teeth through the years. As her friend had described, the experience was not physically painful or embarrassing. She has since gotten over her fear and has adopted healthy dental habits, a path she is sure to continue on that for the rest of her life. Sandy was a perfect candidate for sedation dentistry because all she really required was emotional support combined with physical comfort.

Nitrous Oxide or Laughing Gas

Most commonly, dentists today use nitrous oxide or laughing gas. First used in the 1800s, laughing gas provides light sedation during treatment, making the process more bearable.

On the plus side, nitrous oxide alleviates patient discomfort and exits the body quickly, leaving no lingering side effects. Unfortunately, this treatment also has some major negative attributes: for one thing, it's not very powerful, so it doesn't really do much for most dental patients. For patients who, on their first visit, won't even let a dentist look in their mouth, more substantial help is needed. Laughing gas can help the slightly phobic patients, but for those with severe fears, the nitrous oxide does very little to help. These highly phobic patients are at a whole different level, one that nitrous oxide cannot touch.

Plus, research has shown some concern over the substance. One study in Sweden, which evaluated the effectiveness of nitrous oxide over the last 200 years, led the anesthesiology department at the University Erlangen-Nürnberg to discontinue its traditional use completely.

The major concern with nitrous oxide is overdosing. Too high a percentage of nitrous will deprive the brain of oxygen potentially leading to serious life-threatening consequences. Dental offices that utilize nitrous oxide are not required by law to monitor a patient's oxygen levels, which can lead to serious complications. Nausea, intestinal and ear pain have also been reported with nitrous oxide use. Nitrous oxide should not be given to pregnant women as it has been shown to lead to birth defects and premature labor.

However, if used correctly in healthy patients, nitrous oxide is generally considered to be safe and can be used to ease mild forms of anxiety.

Oral Sedatives or Sleeping Pills

Oral sedatives or sleeping pills are often used to treat patients with dental phobias. Oral sedative pills are given to the patient one to two hours before treatment; this pill makes some patients groggy and actually puts others to sleep. For patients with needle phobia, for example, oral premedication with benzodiazepines or other antianxiety agents can help patients avoid hypotension, unconsciousness, convulsions, and other demonstrations of fear.

At the same time though, oral sedatives have their limits. One of the biggest issues is they can't be titrated (i.e., customized in measurements to suit a patient's specific situation and needs). Since the right dosage isn't only based on a patient's height or weight, it's hard to know how much is necessary to effectively cover them through treatment. An extremely anxious individual may need a higher dose to produce relaxation. However, too large of a dose will put a patient dangerously deep in sedation. If a patient is too heavily sedated, respiratory function can diminish and protective reflexes will be gone. This can be very dangerous, especially in light of the fact that oral medication cannot be reversed quickly if needed. If too low of a dosage is given, adequate sedation may not be achieved and the patient will need to take more pills, wait additional hours for the medication to sink in, and try again.

The Instant Solution for Dental Phobic Patients

The Miracle of IV Sedation

Patients who won't even let dentists look in their mouths have severe dental phobias. Therapy can be a way to treat this condition. While therapy can produce fantastic results, it does take time. Unfortunately, a majority of dental phobic patients have immediate dental needs, active infection, multiple missing teeth, and other problems. These patients need the care of dentists that offer IV sedation, which is a highly specialized treatment option custom designed for phobic patients.

IV sedation is common in oral surgery offices. Many times, unfortunately, patients find themselves in an oral surgeon's office when their situation is beyond restorability. At that point, an oral surgeon will address the chief complaint and, more often than not, remove teeth using IV sedation or general anesthesia. Although this approach will likely alleviate a patient's pain, it is not the ideal approach. The correct approach to this situation would be to have a comprehensive plan of restoration of teeth before extraction in a comfortable setting. This type of plan can be achieved with a group of dental specialists combined with IV sedation. Many phobic patients are not aware that this type of service exists.

Ideal dental treatment for phobic patients consists of

both IV sedation and a specialist approach to treating complex dental problems. Dental specialists such as prosthodontists, periodontists, and endodontists are uniquely trained to treat complex dental problems properly and efficiently. When performed under IV sedation, procedures are done correctly, in total comfort, and with little memory of the actual treatment. Past negative dental incidents are replaced with positive experiences, giving patients hope for a fearless and healthy dental future.

The beauty of IV sedation is that it is administered directly through an IV, so when the patient wakes up, everything is all done. They don't have to be aware of the treatment or feel the anticipated pain they're so afraid of. Instead, patients wake up and say, "Wow, what time is it?" And they can't believe their treatment is already completed. They say, "You did all that already?"

Sharon's Story
Overcoming Dental Phobia in One Visit

As an example of how this works, there is Sharon— a patient who came from an affluent family and had been given just about everything while she was growing up. As she had aged, she'd started getting into designer prescription drug abuse, and eventually, she was a full-on drug addict, having to go through rehabilitation. By the time she found her way to seeking dental care, she was at a halfway house.

At Sharon's first dental visit, she was crying hysteri-

cally. She couldn't face the dentist; her smile was in very bad shape from the drug abuse, and she was extremely embarrassed, with very low self-esteem from all she'd been through.

Extreme dental pain forced Sharon to seek treatment, but she was still afraid. Her family lived out of town, so the social worker from the halfway house escorted her to the appointment.

Right away, it was obvious that treating Sharon's problems would not be easy. Even getting her in the chair was difficult. She was very afraid and reluctant; yet, she also knew she needed the treatment. The dentists got the sedation started, and while she rested in peaceful twilight, they did a lot of work without causing her the slightest discomfort. She had a number of root canal treatments, several extractions, implants placed, some fillings—and she did great. After just that first visit, her smile was already looking good. She woke up, amazed at what had been accomplished, and she was thankful to look better so quickly. Anyone could see that her self-esteem was rising.

After that initial visit, Sharon did need to return for more dental care, but every time it got a little easier. On her second visit, she wasn't crying, but was still a little nervous. With each successive visit, she grew less afraid and more pleased with the results of looking and feeling so much better. It was the IV sedation that allowed her to be able to undergo all of the treatment.

Fast-forward until she was totally done with all her

treatments, and Sharon was a completely different woman. She walked into the office on her own and said, "You know, I don't even need sedation anymore." Talk about a transformation!

Sharon's story is one of the biggest success stories regarding IV sedation. Through the comfort level IV sedation was able to provide, Sharon was totally transformed and conquered her dental fears. Now, she looks fantastic and her self-confidence is high. She started out feeling so low, but now anyone can see that she is well on the path to a successful and constructive life.

For Sharon and many other patients, transforming their smiles played a major role in transforming their lives. The IV sedation made it possible: it nearly cured these nervous patients of their previous dental fears and anxieties. Now, Sharon is all set to maintain her new smile with regular visits to the dentist. She's so pleased with the results that she's even been referring friends.

IV Sedation Dentistry as a Form of Behavioral Therapy

Sedation dentistry also makes it possible for a patient to begin treatment knowing that they will not be judged or made to feel embarrassed. A gentle environment, combined with IV sedation, allows the patient to ease back into visiting the dentist. The dental office will become a source of comfort rather than a source of fear and pain. Following each visit, the patient leaves the office with a good memory and an already significant improvement in their dental health. Many patients reach a point in which the sedation is not necessary at all, though it is always available.

The role that Respiratory Sinus Arrhythmia (RSA) plays so successfully in the treatment of phobias using virtual reality is almost identical to the role that IV sedation plays in dentistry. Both are extremely relaxing and pleasurable, serving the desired dual purpose of generating the conscious experience of counter conditioning and desensitization. This allows the patient's emotional state, in relation to visiting the dentist, to be altered sufficiently to result in the phobia's disappearance.

The reason that IV sedation has been successful for patients with dental phobias (where general anesthesia has failed), is that while under IV sedation the patient retains consciousness (albeit a depressed state). The unconscious state associated with general anesthesia makes any exposure to the feared situation impossible, while IV sedation allows gradual exposure. In other words, the type of learning that seems to be required for successful desensitization can be accomplished while in the twilight state experienced with IV sedation, but not while under general anesthesia.

Sedation Dentistry With CBT for Extreme Dental Phobia

The Combined Approach

For the extremely phobic patient just scheduling the appointment may be an impossible task. In these cases, starting out with CBT in which the therapist uses biofeedback and VRT can be extremely useful. The patient will use the skills he has mastered in practice in the therapist's office to relax for the actual appointment. This will allow the patient to experience minimal stress leading up to and during the dental appointment.

At the conclusion of the first dental appointment, it is likely that the experience will be such that anxiety levels related to visiting the dentist will automatically be reduced. The delicate nature of sedation dentistry is likely to lead to the reduction of anxiety. When necessary, combining the tools learned in CBT to combat anxiety with sedation dentistry makes it is possible for the dental experience to be virtually anxiety free, even for the most phobic patients. With these treatments available, everyone, including people who were once terrified to visit the dentist, can finally regain the feeling of being in control of their lives.

Jake's Story:

Severe Dental Phobia
Psychological Therapy Prior to
Sedation Dentistry

Jake had not been to the dentist for many years. Although he knew he had some strange stuff going on in his mouth, he couldn't get himself to actually make an appointment. He had done research on the internet and learned about sedation dentistry and liked the idea. He hated the thought of numerous office visits over a long period of time. The fact that sedation dentistry would allow him to get the majority of the work done in one visit was appealing to him. He even asked his physician for a referral to a dentist specializing in sedation dentistry and was given one who was highly recommended.

Every time he thought about scheduling the appointment he became extremely anxious and couldn't get himself to make the call. He flossed all the time and brushed religiously as a means to extend the time he could go before actually going to the dentist. He knew he was only avoiding the inevitable. He was impressed by everything he read about sedation therapy but still couldn't bring himself to making the initial appointment. If just making the call was so difficult, how would he ever get himself to the office and into the dental chair?

One night when he was up with a toothache he spent hours researching dental phobias on the internet. That same night he learned about the CBT method of combining biofeedback with virtual reality therapy in treating phobias. In desperation, he hoped that this was what he needed to prepare himself for his first visit to the dentist.

After a few weekly sessions with a CBT therapist, Jake and his psychologist decided he was ready for sedation dentistry. Using the referral he had received from his physician, Jake made the appointment from his therapist's office. He was able to use the RSA breathing technique he had been taught, prior to making the call and before and during his initial visit. Even today, Jake finds the breathing very helpful in reducing stress in many areas of his life. He no longer worries so much about waking up at four o'clock in the morning with thoughts spinning out of control because he now manages them via RSA breathing.

Jake got through his first appointment and is relieved he can smile without shame. Few people can understand what a difference this makes in a their life. CBT combined with sedation dentistry was just what Jake needed to conquer his debilitating phobia. He continues to use the breathing he learned to relax for his regular cleaning, but finds sedation no longer a necessity.

What to Expect from IV Sedation

With IV sedation, patients experience complete relaxation while their dentists work. They have pleasant dreams and the time flies by. When it's over, they have no memory of any of the procedures and, when they leave their appointment, they are happy.

This is so important because it shows that IV sedation offers a way to counteract even the most severe fears. Patients who initially wouldn't even let dentists look in their mouths turn into patients giving thumbs up and saying, "Wow, that was amazing."

It is also important to note that IV sedation is not the same thing as general anesthesia. In general anesthesia, patients lose their protective reflexes and often need assistance to maintain respiratory function. With IV sedation on the other hand, patients maintain their reflexes and are able to breathe on their own. Because of its efficacy and lower risk, IV sedation is becoming widely used for a whole scope of medical procedures, such as certain plastic surgeries, colonoscopies, minor gynecological procedures, and many other outpatient procedures.

IV sedation consists of medication(s) administered intravenously. It works instantaneously, and it produces complete relaxation. Patients under IV sedation rest in "twilight" and dream peacefully while their dentists complete their work. Their fears are abated and their smiles are restored, and even the most complicated work can be done in just a few hours.

Under IV sedation, patients are not aware of the dental procedures being performed. They feel like they're in a happy, relaxed place, where all of their previous dental fears and anxieties just float away. When they wake up, it seems like all the work took place in a matter of minutes, and they can leave feeling good and comfortable, in a very pleasant state.

IV Sedation Can Be Titrated

Because every person is different, titration is very important. Titration is the process by which dentists determine the right concentration of sedation to use, based on a patient's individual characteristics and needs. The sedation is administered in a precise dose, keeping the patient fully sedated without the dangers of going too deep. Where with other forms of sedation (such as oral sedatives or sleeping pills) it can be very hard to predict the amount needed for one individual, IV sedation can be fully titrated.

IV Sedation Is Low Risk

While IV sedation provides patients with complete relaxation and comfort, patients do not lose their ability to breathe on their own and respond to verbal commands. This is a big advantage because although patients won't remember much about the procedure, all factors that could make them nervous or anxious are eliminated. The state of twilight relaxation and the fact that the procedures will seem to be over very quickly help ease virtually all dental fear and anxiety.

IV sedation dentists will offer this wonderful service to patients who want or need to take advantage of it, but they will also offer other options. Typically, it seems that about 90 percent of phobic patients will opt to take advantage of IV sedation when it's available. This is why specialty practices that offer this sedation method are highly skilled and sought after by patients from all over the country.

Dental Work Done in the Blink of an Eye

During a period of just a few hours, dentists can accomplish a lot of work. It's amazing what total transformations can take place in one short window of time. That's one of the biggest advantages of IV sedation: it makes it possible to do all that work in one brief, condensed visit.

Even patients who are unafraid of dental treatment may still choose IV sedation because it provides a way to rest peacefully in twilight while a great deal of work is accomplished. With specialty dental offices that offer IV sedation, it is possible to enjoy a painless, stress-free, treatment that is over in the blink of an eye. Anyone who has had dental procedures done this way will tell you that it's a much better way to go to the dentist.

Jeffrey's Story

Jeffrey is an example of a patient who wasn't afraid of the dentist but still benefited from IV sedation. As someone who started having treatments without sedation, Jeffrey felt like everything was going fine. He was not fearful, but because his dentists needed to do so many treatments, he opted to try sedation. After he tried it, he said, "Oh, I don't want to go back. I don't want to be in the chair and actively participate when I could be relaxing! I want to rest and wake up when everything's done."

Even though Jeffrey knew he had nothing to be afraid of and had previously undergone many procedures without sedation, he still realized it was much less stress on him to be sedated.

Undergoing treatments with or without sedation is always the patient's choice. Some need it, some want it, and some are relieved to try it. Whatever the case, unique practices that offer it are providing a rare opportunity to make dental treatments simpler, easier, and more comfortable.

Misconceptions of Sedation

Is It Safe?

There are many misconceptions of IV sedation. Many people wonder if it is safe—it is. In order to become certified in IV sedation, dentists must successfully complete intensive training in Anesthesia and Sedation. IV sedation dentists must also complete advanced training in medical emergencies and receive a special license from the State or governmental agency. Before any patient undergoes IV sedation, dentists are required take a very thorough medical history to make sure that the person is healthy enough to handle it. Then, during any procedure where a patient is sedated, the dentists are legally required to monitor the patient's vital signs, watching pulse, blood pressure, oxygen saturation, and electrocardiogram (EKG) constantly. Plus, there will be emergency equipment available in the very unlikely event that it would be needed. Complications are rare during sedation, but good dentists will be prepared for anything.

The truth is, when administered by a trained and experienced specialist, IV sedation is very safe. One of the reasons it is so appealing is because there are effective reversal agents for many of the medications typically used in IV sedation. Dentists can actually reverse the effects of the sedation instantaneously. For example, if they start noticing a concerning dip in any vital signs, they can reverse the sedation immediately. As such, IV sedation is safer than other forms of anesthesia.

Is It Reliable?

IV sedation is also very predictable compared to other forms of anesthesia. By using a combination of medications, the sedation specialist can use the needed amount to create a desired sedative effect.

Are There Any Restrictions Before and After IV Sedation?

One of the most common questions regarding IV sedation is whether patients will be able to drive themselves to and from their appointments. The answer is no; patients should plan to be driven to and from their treatments because some lingering effects of the sedation could make it unsafe to drive immediately following their appointments. Additionally, patients should not eat or drink for about four hours prior to sedation. If a patient is taking prescription medicine, it is important for the sedation specialist to discuss the situation and planned treatment beforehand with the patient's physician.

How Will I Feel?

Prospective patients are also often curious about how they will feel during the sedation. The simple answer is relaxed, unaware of what's going on, and comfortable. Afterwards, patients might be a little groggy; however, the most common medications used are short-acting, so the after-effects dissipate pretty quickly.

It's also important to mention that everybody reports the same thing. During sedation, a long dental visit feels like it was completed in a few short minutes. Time passes very quickly, making the treatment even more comfortable and painless.

Is IV Sedation Common in Dental Offices?

IV sedation in dental offices offering comprehensive treatment isn't common at all. This service is much more common for oral surgery procedures, such as tooth extractions. However, patients who require complex dental work are in need of various procedures other than tooth extractions. These patients need to do a thorough search to find a group of dental specialists that not only provides IV sedation but also can restore their smile to the highest standards.

Will I Lose Control of My Mind and Body under IV Sedation?

People often think that they will lose control when they are sedated. That is not true. Usually, sedated patients are calm and relaxed, as if they were sleeping. Sometimes patients will come out of the sedation and they will ask, "What did I say?" or "How was I? How did I behave?" Patients worry that they might give too much information or say something embarrassing, but sedation is not a truth serum. People are afraid they will tell all of their secrets, but nobody ever does.

People affected by the sedation are still in control of their breathing and natural reflexes, but they are completely relaxed and do not have any anxiety. The IV sedation creates an atmosphere for them that makes it pleasant to be in a dental chair.

After the positive experience that sedation creates for them, a lot of patients see their lifelong dental fears disappear. They no longer associate the dental chair with pain and fear. For other patients, even if the fear might not completely disappear, it still lessens considerably.

For many people, IV sedation is the most effective way to overcome dental fear; without it, they might never have courage to undergo treatment. Not only does IV sedation allow patients to have much needed dentistry, but it also erases their fear of dentistry.

As all these very phobic patients progress through treatment and when they come back afterwards for follow-ups, they are doing much better psychologically. Previously afraid to let dentists even look in their mouths, they will accept minor adjustments with metal tools with little to no fear. It's the kind of thing they never thought was possible but really happens.

Tanya's Story

When Tanya first came in, she wouldn't even let the dentist look at her. She was so fearful and anxious, even a touch would cause tears. After comprehensive treatment with IV sedation, Tanya returned every six months for her check-up and when it came time for her to need a new dental crown, she was able to have the work done without any sedation. She wasn't afraid anymore—what caused the transformation? She had come so far. It was all because of the difference IV sedation made. SShe trusted her dentists, who had built significant rapport with her and became like friends because of the quality of their treatment. That is how dental procedures should be.

Many patients haven't experienced a nice smile and oral health in decades, so effective treatment becomes a truly life-changing journey. The look of their mouths is something they previously couldn't control, but after overcoming dental fear, they obtain the treatment they need to restore their smile, oral health, and self-esteem.

Fear of Needles

Society has helped build this strong fear of dentists—
and along with it, the fear of needles. Many patients fear
both. For this reason, although most anxious patients
want to take advantage of IV sedation, sometimes they
first must overcome the fear of needles which provide
the sedation.

There is good news. Most of the time, patients who
are afraid of needles are most afraid of needles in the
mouth, and because the IV needle is not placed in the
mouth, it is not as frightening.

But for those patients who are truly afraid of all needles,
there are other options. Before the IV line is started, the
patient could receive a little nitrous oxide to help take
the edge off. A skin refrigerant, a little coolant spray
put right on the skin just before the IV injection, can
help mask the pinch of the needle; this way, patients
really don't feel the needle at all. The IV sedation kicks
in right away, and patients will not even remember the
IV needle.

Dana's Story

IV Sedation & Needle Phobia

*Dana was a patient who was initially very apprehen-
sive about the IV needle. She had extreme dental fear,
created by negative past childhood experiences, sensitivity to being touched in the mouth, and fear of personal space invasion. When she was told the IV would*

be placed in her hand, she wanted avoid treatment entirely. In her case, extra measures were necessary to make it possible for her to receive the IV sedation. She was given nitrous oxide (laughing gas) as well as a light oral sedative to help her relax enough to receive the sedation and undergo necessary treatment in comfort. A skin refrigerant was also used, and the IV was placed without any discomfort or apprehension.

How to Take Control of Your Smile

Taking control of your smile is pretty simple, no matter what your preconceptions or experiences have been. Through IV sedation, any healthy person can undergo treatment in a relaxed state, with no memory of what has happened. Time goes by very quickly.

Bob's Story

A good-looking man with a high-profile job at a law firm in New York City, Bob was an otherwise very successful individual who was walking around with a totally non-functional denture. He wore a purposefully long mustache to camouflage his teeth, that's how socially painful the condition of his smile was for him. Then he found the dentists who could help him. Through eight dental implants, IV sedation, and the skill of a highly specialized team, Bob walked out with teeth that don't move and look great—after one visit. Needless to say, he was thrilled. Shortly thereafter,

84

Bob shaved his mustache and was able to smile proudly in public. He was finally able to go to his favorite restaurant and order whatever he wanted, as opposed to ordering what his denture would allow him to eat.

CHAPTER 6

The Inner Beauty of an Outward Smile

Dental fear, anxiety, and general embarrassment over unattractive teeth prevent many people from scheduling and attending recommended regular dental visits, eventually causing an unhealthy smile. Left untreated, gum disease will take over and that is a serious problem, not just for your mouth but also for your entire body.

Restore the Health of Your Mouth and Live a Longer, Fuller Life

Many patients don't realize how much the health of the mouth affects the rest of the body. A tooth infection can easily spread into surrounding tissues, leading to abscess, swelling, fever, and in extreme cases even death. That's why one of the biggest priorities in proper dental treatment is disinfecting and preventing reinfection. If you can eradicate gum disease infection that causes bad breath and tooth loss, you'll also reduce your risk of heart disease, diabetes, and cancer. One way to do this is through skilled treatment, which will restore your mouth to a healthy state.

Appearance and Health

Everyone knows the power of a beautiful smile: it's one of the first things strangers notice about you and one of the key factors in making a good initial impression. Missing permanent teeth takes away the confidence and comfort of a gorgeous grin by breaking apart the symmetry your mouth was designed to have.

That's why it's so important for patients to be given a personal, customized, revolutionary solution that can solve their unique set of dental challenges. Regardless of the issues treated, all patients should be able to leave the dental office after their first visits with a healthier, aesthetically pleasing smile, looking years younger and feeling confident.

A Nice Smile Is Priceless

There are countless books nowadays that discuss how you can change your life by thinking positively. The books talk about how, by behaving in a positive manner, you can change your life.

Interestingly enough, the easiest way to behave positively is to smile. In fact, many of those books and the psychologists writing them will tell you to remind yourself to smile. Smiling is at the root of behaving positively. You just can't do it without smiling. If you are ashamed to smile or hide your smile, how can you change your life? The very act of smiling can be painful and evoke a whole range of negative emotions.

In order to practice the positivity of smiling, a person

needs a smile that he or she can be proud of, or at least be willing to show. If the condition of your teeth and gums is preventing you from smiling, there is hope. Through proper treatment, you can restore your smile, making you confident to smile at the world. It's a decision that will change your life.

Each month or year that you wait to do something about your teeth is another month or year lost. The value of your investment decreases with each day that slips away. Your new smile will last a lifetime, and the longer you wait, the less you can smile confidently and the longer you have to hide your smile.

A nice smile is truly priceless. It's not about the teeth or the implants or veneers. It's about something much deeper. You can't put a price on your self-esteem and living your life to the fullest. You can't put a price on a beautiful smile—it's something that changes your life.

The point at which you decide to restore your smile will be a pivotal turning point for you. With each passing year, a certain portion of your life will pass, bringing down the value of your investment. Comprehensive treatment will still benefit you, but doing it when you're younger lets you reap the greatest benefits. You'll have fewer bad habits to break, fewer negative experiences to get over.

The sooner you realize that you don't smile because your smile isn't in good condition, the sooner you should do something about it. You will be able to change your life earlier, eliminate bad habits quicker, live your life to the fullest sooner, and enjoy your investment for longer. You can't put a price on that. Don't wait for a catalyst. The time is now.

Imagine This...

Ask anyone who's insecure about his or her smile: changing the look of your teeth can become so important that it's the only thing you think about. The good news is that if you're reading this, you've already taken the first step. Through a *power smile consultation* with dental specialists, you will have made the next step. Once you see how attainable a beautiful smile can be, you will know what you need to do and what journey you want and need to take. It can be easy and comfortable—and it will change your life.

So, imagine this: a complete makeover of your entire look, with whitening, veneers, and all kinds of tweaks— done in just a few hours. By reclaiming your smile, you no longer have to feel or look old due to unattractive or non-functional teeth. In one afternoon, you can regain your confidence and feel younger. There is no waiting for your smile. You simply come in for treatment and leave the same day with a brand-new smile—one that is as functional and healthy as it is beautiful.

Look Younger and Be Healthier

White, attractive looking teeth are typically associated with youth, health, and beauty; so when a patient gets a new, healthier smile, that often leads to a new, healthier life. An attractive appearance causes changes that extend to all kinds of other areas. Whether it's smoking, dieting, or making healthier choices, patients often realize that feeling good about their teeth makes them feel good about themselves, too. Plus, people who feel good about themselves tend to live longer—so a new smile is more than just aesthetic, it can also be the ticket to enjoying more of life.

A New Smile Is Just the Beginning

Having a beautiful smile changes everything. Take smoking: Comprehensive dental treatment can certainly help smokers obtain a whiter, healthier smile, but it can also give them the encouragement to quit altogether. Smoking can cause gum disease and dry mouth, which can lead to cavities and decay, and the habit also definitely worsens gum disease for those who already have it. With new laws discouraging smoking and more research revealing just how bad smoking is for people's health, every single smoker seems to be trying to quit.

What many people don't know is that a new smile is a powerful motivator for kicking the smoking habit. Looking good and feeling energized are positive experiences for anyone, but especially for smokers, as having new, healthy teeth can be just the push they need to quit. For most smokers, a new smile feels like a new lease on life—and choosing to stop smoking is a convenient side effect.

In other cases, new teeth motivate people to move towards other changes, whether diet, exercise, or weight loss. Because a new smile is so powerful, it can be a catalyst for all kinds of positive results. It happens all the time. With a new smile, it feels like anything is possible: that's why a new smile is just the beginning.

Enhanced Quality of Life and Increased Confidence

You can experience an enhanced quality of life with natural-looking teeth designed to appear, feel, and perform just as beautifully as if you were born with them. You don't have to let dentures, missing teeth, or unattractive teeth keep you from experiencing the best life possible. You can be proud of your smile and smile freely and often.

Has a lack of confidence over your smile held you back from something in life? A promotion? More sales? A dating life? It doesn't have to be that way. Getting a brand-new smile may sound too good to be true, but thousands of patients who have experienced the care of dental specialists know it isn't.

They've shaved their mustaches for good. They've stopped hiding their smiles and have been proud to show them off. They are out in the world, getting what they want out of life. You can look better, feel better, improve your love life, fast-track your career, and find motivation to be healthier, whether you're 25 or 50, single or divorced, a parent or a grandparent. It's as simple as a few easy hours in a dental office.

A new, beautiful smile means confidence, increased energy, motivation to move forward, and inspiration to pursue dreams. It means looking great and feeling great. It means being ready to find a new partner to share life with. It means living the life you've always wanted.

Brian's Story

Brian was the typical unhappy middle-aged man, stuck in a rut that he thought he couldn't get out of. When he came in for dental care, he was in a bad marriage where he felt unloved, unappreciated, and in many ways abused. Because his smile was so unattractive, however, he never had the courage to leave his wife. Only after receiving a full mouth reconstruction, which drastically improved his appearance and revolutionized his confidence level, he decided to do something about it. He filed for a divorce because he was no longer afraid. His new smile gave him a new perspective and a new level of courage that nothing else could.

Regardless of your current situation, you are guaranteed to benefit from a new smile and the accompanying happiness it brings. Imagine a life without embarrassment over ugly, yellow, discolored, unattractive, missing, broken, or decayed teeth. Imagine looking in the mirror and loving what you see. With the right specialized approach, these dreams aren't just dreams; they're reality.

Turn Back the Hands of Time

Bad Teeth Make You Look Older

A healthy and beautiful smile is one of the defining attributes of youth. That's why without one—but with an unattractive smile in its place—a person can actually look older and less desirable. The longer the mouth is left unhealthy or with missing teeth, the more deterioration of healthy tissue that will be experienced. Missing teeth can also cause fine lines and wrinkles to develop around the mouth, amplifying the aging process. In fact, because the teeth provide support for the muscles and skin around the mouth, missing teeth result in a loss of support, causing unnecessary stress on those muscles and the skin.

This is a factor that can accelerate the formation of fine lines and wrinkles around the mouth, making a person look older, just like infection in the mouth can seriously jeopardize your overall health, making you look significantly older than you actually are. Without teeth, the bones in the jaw start to deteriorate and resorb. Cheeks look sunken in. Your face starts taking the appearance of somebody who is ten to twenty years older than you are.

Clearly, a smile is about much more than appearances; it's about health, confidence, and making the most of life. Over time, there have been a number of patients who evidenced success in many areas, from careers and finances to family situations, but yet for one reason or another, they didn't take care of their smiles. If they only understood how attainable a beautiful smile can be, they could have take control in this area too, improving their lives and effectively turning back the hands of time.

The Power of First Impressions

In a society where first impressions mean so much, it is important to have a nice smile. The smile is one of the first things someone will notice about you, and if you don't appear to be happy or confident, that can give a negative first impression. Moreover, it has been researched and reported that even babies respond much better to people who smile and who have a nice healthy smile. It's innate.

Katie's Story

Very attractive and obviously well pulled together, Katie was a 45 year old woman that had a lot going for her. Nonetheless, when she stepped into a dental office, she looked gloomy and unhappy; she couldn't even greet the woman at the front desk with a smile. This was typical for Katie. She didn't mean to seem unfriendly, but she'd been ashamed of her smile for so long, she'd gotten used to not smiling. By behaving this way, she had projected the image that was a complete opposite of who she really was. If you got to know her, you'd see she had a wonderful personality and a fantastic sense of humor that made her a pleasure to speak with. But unfortunately, unless you got to know her, she gave the strong impression of being a mean, nasty woman, one with a continually negative facial expression that had become a habit over the years as she tried to hide her teeth. She said she spent most of her life working to overcome that first impression—and the worst part was she did not even know what was causing it.

After finishing dental treatment, Katie got her smile back and learned how to use it again. Finally, her expressions matched her personality and people could easily see what a great person she was. And thankfully, Katie found, it takes much less time to learn to smile than to learn not to smile. It's easy to get used to a good thing!

"*A woman whose smile is open and whose expression is glad has a kind of beauty no matter what she wears.*"
— Anne Roiphe

CHAPTER 7

Dental Procedures

As mentioned earlier in this book, many people who suffer from Dental Phobia have a fear of the unknown. The mere thought of sitting in a dental chair with the piercing sound of the high speed drill causes extreme anxiety and apprehension. In the preceding chapters, several treatment alternatives have been offered, from psychotherapy to Sedation Dentistry, with the goal of physiologically reducing dental anxiety. The aim of the following chapter is to explain some of the modern day dental treatments. By having an understanding of the pain free procedures and technologies that dentists utilize in reversing and treating dental problems, patients can reduce their "fear of the unknown". This can lead to the positive realization that many procedures can be done both comfortably and quickly.

Restoring Teeth

Think of dental restorations as you would any other restoring process. Whether it involves cleaning a room, repainting walls, or refinishing furniture, a restoration aims to bring things back to their original quality. This is exactly the case with your teeth.

Dental restorations become necessary for a variety of reasons, not just because of caries. Other common causes include accidents or trauma, erosion of enamel from a highly acidic diet, toothbrush abrasion, congenital anomalies, and even cosmetic needs. Whatever the reason, dental restorations are very important for preventing further decay, as well as for improving both comfort and appearance for patients. Today, there are many types of restorations available, depending upon your given needs.

Caries

Though the terms are often used interchangeably, caries and cavities are not exactly the same thing. Caries actually refers to the disease process that leads to cavities.

Cause of Caries

Essentially, the cause of caries goes back to bacteria called *Streptococcus mutans*. In a patient with caries, these bacteria get nourishment from sugar in food, allowing them to produce acids, make plaque and form cavities, eventually causing a need for restorations.

Because bacteria grow by latching onto the sugar left in your mouth from certain foods, a nutritious diet is key in eliminating caries. Simply cutting back on high-sugar items such as sticky candy, sugary cereals, soft drinks, and other high-sugar beverages makes a dramatic difference in your oral health.

Three things are necessary for a cavity to develop:

- **High-sugar foods left in mouth:** It's not just the food but also the duration! The longer sugar sits on the teeth, the more damage it can do.

- **Host response:** The bacteria in your mouth can trigger an immune response from your body. Your body's cells are trying to fight the bacteria, and sometimes a person's own cells can damage teeth and gums.

- **Bad oral hygiene:** Without the preventative maintenance of proper oral care, the bacteria can run rampant and develop fully into a cavity.

When these three factors combine, cavities form, leading to a variety of complications, from discomfort and pain to restorations.

Reasons for Restorations

Typically, when people think of reasons for restorations, they think of caries, and it's true that caries is one of the main causes. However, caries is just one of many causes for restoration work, including trauma, erosion of enamel, toothbrush abrasion, congenital anomalies, and cosmetic needs. Restoration is a way of replacing missing or lost structure, both for functional and aesthetic purposes.

Trauma

Whether brought on by a sporting injury, a car accident, or some other kind of violence, dental trauma often requires restoration. Sometimes this involves, for example, repairing a cracked tooth with a filling or a crown. Other times, it may mean reinserting a tooth that's been knocked out.

There are steps you can take to avoid dental trauma, even beyond practicing good oral hygiene and visiting the dentist regularly. Especially if you are involved in strenuous physical activity, you may wish to wear a custom mouth guard created by your dentist.

Erosion of Enamel

When the thin outer layer of teeth—enamel—erodes, a tooth loses its strongest protector. This exposes the nerves, leading to increased sensitivity to hot and cold temperatures, discomfort, pain, and sometimes a need for restorations. One of the leading causes for this erosion is a high-acid diet, filled with soft drinks and fruit drinks with phosphoric and citric acids.

Eating Disorders

There are also other more serious causes of enamel

erosion, ranging from gastrointestinal disease to eating disorders like bulimia nervosa and anorexia nervosa. If a patient suffers from bulimia nervosa, for example, he or she regularly binges on food and then vomits in order to control weight gain. One of the many damaging effects of this constant vomiting is that it forces stomach acids into the mouth and thus against the teeth, leading to enamel erosion. Anorexia nervosa leads to both enamel erosion, as well as improper caries response, due to abnormal carbohydrate consumption.

Acid Reflux Disorder

What happens in acid reflux disorder is a continual reflux of stomach contents and acids into the oral cavity causes major loss of tooth structure.

Usually hard to detect and diagnose, acid reflux disorder often causes severe enamel erosion by the time a patient realizes he or she has the disorder. That's why early detection by a dentist can be vital not just in treatment and restoration, but also in prevention.

Toothbrush Abrasion

Like erosion, toothbrush abrasion wears away the tooth's outer coating of enamel. It happens when a patient brushes too hard (often with a hard-bristled brush), or when something scrapes against the teeth. A toothbrush isn't the only culprit in this type of abrasion; toothpicks may also damage the teeth, as well as removable devices like partial dentures or retainers. You will know if you have toothbrush abrasion by looking at the bottom third of your teeth, close to the gums: check for V-shaped marks right in or between teeth.

Cosmetic Reasons

For many people, more attractive teeth make all the difference in how they feel about their overall appearance. Restorations provide a way to achieve that perfect smile through a variety of treatments, such as filling in gaps between teeth, for example, both because it's more visually pleasing and because it helps prevent food impaction.

Bonding is a specific restoration that improves tooth appearance. In this process, tooth-colored composite resin gets bonded to teeth, which is ideal for closing small gaps. Its beautiful results usually last around five to seven years. For more on bonding, see the chapter on cosmetic dentistry.

Anatomy of a Tooth

To really understand the way restorations work, it is helpful to take a look at the basic structure of your teeth. While we are all familiar with the shape and color of teeth, there's actually a lot more at work.

Three of the basic components of a tooth are enamel, dentin, and pulp.

- **Enamel:** The outermost layer of a tooth is a hard, white, translucent substance called enamel. Strong and durable enough to stand up against all the chewing and biting you do on a regular basis, enamel is still easy to crack. Unlike bones, enamel doesn't repair easily, and that's why taking care of it is so important.

- **Dentin**: Beneath enamel, dentin is a softer substance that makes up the majority of the tooth. While coffee, tea, and poor oral hygiene can stain enamel, the most common teeth stains stem from the dentin. Certain diseases, too much fluoride, or even aging can change the shade of the dentin, making teeth look discolored.

- **Pulp**: The middle layer of a tooth is the pulp (or root canal), which houses blood vessels and nerves that feel sensations of temperature and pain.

When Decay Deepens

As decay goes deeper into the heart of a tooth, a filling becomes larger, increasing the chances of the tooth breaking. In some cases, this means a crown has to be fitted over what's left of the tooth. If the decay extends all the way into the pulp/nerve, a root canal may even be necessary to avoid losing the tooth completely.

Where Cavities Occur

The reality is that cavities can occur on several different surfaces of the tooth, and there are a variety of treatments available, depending upon the extent of decay. In early stages, cavities are best treated with fillings, which can be placed on any surface.

Q: How can I tell if I have a cavity?

A: Depending on how far the decay has spread, you may notice a toothache or increased sensitivity to hot and cold foods or very sweet foods or drinks. It's also possible for cavities to cause visible holes and/or discoloration and dark spots in the teeth. In the early stages (when detection is key), it can be hard to tell: that's why dental checkups are so important. Your dentist can see if a tooth feels soft and/or if X-rays show what is not yet visible.

Early Detection Is Key

When it comes to cavities, the sooner you can catch them, the better. The goal is to spot decay in the very early stages so that it can be stopped and treated, and so that you can keep as much of your tooth as possible.

Remineralization

One hot new area of research in the area of restorations is the noninvasive method of remineralization. According to a recent study, this newer treatment provides an effective way to stop and repair early caries by increasing mineral gain during the normal cycles of demineralization and remineralization.

Essentially, the way remineralization works is this: calcium and phosphate ions get added to the tooth to encourage mineral gain in the weakened enamel.

Rather than merely treating the damage, remineralization offers a way to rebuild what was lost, without any major surgery or painful treatment options.

Crowns, Bridges, Onlays, Inlays

Crowns

Designed to restore appearance and function of teeth that have been thoroughly damaged by decay or trauma, crowns (also called caps) are a common form of restoration. Their name comes from the part of the tooth they cover—the crown or the top—and they are cemented on for durability. When a tooth is almost gone, held together merely by a large filling or so weak that it could break further, a crown serves to prevent further damage and preserve what is there. There are three main types of crowns: full metal, porcelain fused to metal, and all ceramic.

Bridges

In cases where a tooth needs to be replaced, bridgework is one option for restoration. Bridgework involves the creation of prosthetic teeth, which are attached to a crown and then attached to supporting teeth. Usually good for 10 years, bridges provide a reliable way to replace lost or removed teeth, but not all teeth can be replaced this way.

Onlays & Inlays

Specifically made in a laboratory to fit a tooth, onlays and inlays replace lost tooth material. Very costly, these restorations are similar to fillings but larger in size, set into the bumps on the surface of a tooth.

Onlays are larger than inlays, but both can be made of a variety of materials, including gold, composite resin, or ceramics. According to a recent study, ceramic inlays and onlays are particularly beneficial, both in terms of aesthetics and durability, in situations where posterior teeth are especially damaged.

Fillings

Prevention is always the best option in caring for your teeth; however, when decay does occur, fillings offer an effective method for preventing further damage. They help fill in the biting surface of a decayed tooth after all decay has been removed. Fillings are available in four different materials: amalgam, gold, composite, or porcelain, and each has different pluses and minuses to consider.

Take amalgam (sometimes called silver): though shown for over a century to be a successful and cost-effective filling material, this substance has recently created a lot of controversy. From an environmental standpoint, there is concern about the amount of mercury discharged into wastewater from dental offices.

From a health standpoint, there are many who believe the liquid mercury in amalgam can lead to a host of serious medical issues, from multiple sclerosis to hearing loss. Despite these fears, the truth is that no reliable or authoritative studies have been conclusive enough to lead to a national ban on the material. In fact, a 2004 study for the U.S. Public Health Service found "insufficient evidence of a link between dental mercury and health problems, except in rare instances of allergic reaction."

In our generation of prevention, it still makes sense to choose a material you feel most comfortable with; however, the biggest reason we avoid amalgam is a cosmetic one: it's simply not as attractive as other options.

Composite Fillings

The most common alternative to amalgam, composite fillings are white, tooth-colored fillings made from resin reinforced with powdered glass.

Benefits of Composite Fillings

The benefits of composite fillings are aesthetics and convenience. Because of their tooth-colored shade, composite fillings blend right in with other teeth, creating the most attractive restoration. They minimize the amount of healthy tooth removal needed, and they are very convenient, able to be applied in just one dental visit.

Disadvantages of Composite Fillings

Despite the convenience of composite fillings, there are some major problems associated with this material. Composite is very technique-sensitive: any moisture that contacts the material as it sets can negatively affect the integrity of the filling, leading to recurrent decay. Anecdotally, we have seen hundreds of failed composite fillings with such severe recurrent decay that the teeth often need root canals. Additionally, there has been some recent talk of composite fillings leaking bisphenol A (BPA), a chemical shown in animal testing to increase risk for heart health issues, cancer, diabetes, sexual dysfunction, and hyperactivity.

Based on a thorough understanding of composite materials, it is our recommendation that composite only be used in shallow cavities that can be properly isolated during the placement so no moisture gets in, and all of the margins of the filling are accessible and visible to ensure a tight seal.

Gold Fillings

Gold fillings are a durable filling option used to restore decay on a tooth's biting surface. Created from a combination of gold, copper, and other metals, gold alloy has been used for quite a while and doesn't fracture under stress.

Benefits of Gold Fillings

What makes gold fillings a good choice is their time-tested, established use. Gold doesn't corrode in the mouth, and it wears well. Also, as a soft metal, gold conforms to the walls of the filling and causes a stable seal. When gold fillings are fitting properly, they offer excellent resistance to further decay.

Disadvantages of Gold Fillings

The drawbacks of gold fillings are that they have to be made in a lab and require at least two visits to implement, making them inconvenient and costly. They can irritate sensitive teeth, particularly in response to hot and cold because of how the metal conducts temperatures. Additionally, because gold fillings don't match teeth in color but are rather yellow, they are not as aesthetically pleasing as other options.

Porcelain Fillings

A glassy, tooth-colored material, porcelain is yet another filling option. Porcelain fillings are made in a dental lab from an impression and usually reserved for larger fillings such as onlays and inlays.

Benefits of Porcelain Fillings

Porcelain fillings offer beautiful aesthetics with their tooth-colored appearance and customized fit. The new metal-free material lithium disilicate (IPS e.max) offers a fresh take on porcelain fillings. According to a recent study, clinical trials for the last four years have yielded very positive findings regarding this strong and versatile material, which was determined to be one of the best restorative materials available.

Disadvantages of Porcelain Fillings

The downside of porcelain fillings is the cost, as well as the fact that they usually take two visits to implement. However, new digital technology has improved restorations using porcelain tremendously.

New Technology for Porcelain Fillings

The E4D Dentist CAD Cam system and the Chairside Economical Restoration of Esthetic Ceramics (CEREC) porcelain-milling machine are two new developments improving the way porcelain fillings are made.

These systems allow dentists to create restorations right in the office, eliminating the need for an outside dental laboratory and without waiting a long time for a completed product.

Dental offices that offer an in-house E4D or CEREC system can provide patients with same-day turnaround on porcelain crowns, veneers and inlays. This means all the benefits of porcelain fillings—beautiful appearance, easy blend with other teeth, customized fit—without the lengthy wait time or multiple office visits.

Root Canals

At the very mention of a root canal, many people panic. For decades, root canals have had a reputation of being painful, intensive, and terrifying, despite the fact that they're actually made to alleviate pain. Thankfully, root canals don't have to be painful, and, in cases of severe nerve damage, they can make the difference between losing a tooth and keeping it. With IV sedation and the help of an endodontist, a root canal can be performed quickly and painlessly, helping you keep your teeth in the process.

What Is a Root Canal?

A root canal is a treatment that's designed to save a tooth from becoming so damaged it has to be removed. The way it works is this: a dentist takes out dead or dying nerve tissues and bacteria from inside a tooth that's been deeply infected either by a tooth crack, cavity, or some kind of injury, with damage all the way down to the nerves at the root. After removing those nerve tissues, the dentist then cleans and seals the tooth for protection.

Fear of Root Canals

When it comes to dreaded dental treatments, nothing seems to be more feared than the root canal. Horror stories about root canals are everywhere, filled with descriptions of major pain and discomfort. In one study, 35% of respondents anticipated root canal treatment to be the most unpleasant dental procedure, even more so than oral surgery; however, the same study showed that while fear is common in new patients, those who have already experienced a root canal are much less anxious.

That's because the good news is a root canal doesn't have to be difficult. In fact, when done properly and efficiently, it can be an easy experience—one that eliminates the pain and swelling associated with damaged nerves in an infected tooth. In a study of 176 patients who received root canals, over half experienced absolutely no pain at all. Another study showed the likelihood of persistent pain after root canal treatment was only around 5.3%.

Ways to Eliminate Root Canal Anxiety

Clear communication, anesthesia, and other tools can be used to significantly reduce dental anxiety and make the root canal procedure more comfortable.

As is the case with many phobias, understanding what to expect makes a big difference, as it relieves the fear of the unknown. There have even been studies that suggest certain external factors—such as listening to relaxing music through headphones—can make the root canal treatment less frightening and increase patient comfort with the experience.

Mostly though, IV sedation can revolutionize the root canal experience. It makes the time pass quickly and painlessly. Patients rest safely while their mouths are restored to a healthy state, and, best of all, root canals provide a way to keep your natural teeth, which is always the preferable option.

Root Canals Reinvented: The Importance of an Endodontist

Patients should always see an endodontist, even for a simple root canal. An endodontist offers specialized training in performing root canals and so can do multiple root canals, from start to finish, in just one visit. You may think that seems impossible, but the reality is that with a specialist, root canals can truly be done quickly while still being performed properly and efficiently. Furthermore, research has shown patients are more satisfied with treatment performed by an endodontist.

With the best endodontists, root canals aren't only quick but also comfortable, leaving patients smiling when they leave the office. That's why many general dentists refer their patients to endodontists: in one recent study of 220 general dental practitioners in Northern Ireland, for example, 94% referred patients to a specialist endodontist over other treatment providers.

As experienced dental practitioners, endodontists understand the importance of a rubber dam, which can isolate a tooth during a procedure to prevent saliva and other bacteria-heavy fluids from getting inside. While dental students and even many dentists feel that the rubber dam is a hindrance to getting treatment done, the truth is that rubber dams are crucial tools, not only to prevent bacterial contamination but also to prevent the swallowing of small instruments during the procedure. Pediatric dentists use rubber dams either always or frequently in their day-to-day work and consider it a standard of care. However, it's just as important for adult dental work: if your dentist doesn't use a rubber dam, find a new dentist!

Josie's Story

Josie, a young woman who was in need of root canal treatment, came to one of the few endodontists who offered IV sedation to perform her procedures. Her father escorted her to the appointment. During her visit, when Josie had six root canals done, her father commented on being amazed that all the procedures could be finished in one visit. When he had gotten just one root canal performed at his own dentist's office, the process took a total of three visits, with a great deal of drilling back and forth. He couldn't believe the contrast in his daughter's treatment, where so much more could be done in so much less time. That's the benefit of seeing a specialist: they're able to do so much more for you expertly. This means less time in the chair, less discomfort, and a healthy, functional, beautiful smile in the simplest way possible.

If you're thinking that six root canals would be a lot of stress on the body, here's the truth: actually, performing all of the root canals in one visit with IV sedation puts much less stress on the body than doing them just one or two at a time. With this method, the dentists are cleaning up all of the infection quickly. If they were doing just one or two root canals at a time, the patient deals with infection until all the root canals are completed. Plus, the extended time undergoing treatment means extended time dealing with fear, anxiety, and discomfort—putting considerable extra stress on the body.

Dentists can reduce and even eliminate a lot of that stress through IV sedation. Most of the time, patients don't feel or remember much, and that is a good thing. It not only improves the experience for them, but it also helps them recover much more easily.

Gum Disease

In most cases, gum disease is a bacterial infection, afflicting gums and bone around teeth. It may affect one or many teeth, and it grows more serious with time. If left untreated, gum disease will lead to tooth loss and a need for dentures. According to recent findings published in the *Journal of Dental Research*, gum disease is much more common than expected—as much as 50% of adults have some form of gum disease.

In fact, the American Academy of Periodontology estimates that three out of four Americans deal with some form of gum disease, and yet only three percent seek treatment.

Left untreated, gum disease will inevitably take over. The harmful bacteria seep into the gums, destroying teeth, and the infection can spread to other parts of the body and even cause oral cancer or heart disease.

Q: Doesn't everyone lose his or her teeth eventually?

A: You don't have to lose your teeth; they were made to last a lifetime. However, the leading cause of tooth loss in adults 35 and older is untreated periodontal disease. That's why it's so important to stop the disease from progressing and catch it as early as possible.

Stages of Gum Disease

Gum disease is a broad category used to describe the infection of gums, which may begin almost imperceptibly and yet can advance into damage serious enough to cause tooth loss.

Beginning Gum Disease: Gingivitis

Gum disease begins with gingivitis, where the gums are swollen, red, and may bleed. As the mildest form of gum disease, gingivitis causes little, if any, discomfort and is reversible with the right treatment and oral care.

Q: Is it normal for gums to bleed?

A: No. Bleeding gums are one of several warning signs of gum disease, along with swollen or tender gums, oral sores, gums pulling away from teeth, and habitual bad breath. If you notice these symptoms, you should see a dentist.

Advanced Gum Disease: Periodontitis

However, if untreated, gum disease will progress from gingivitis into periodontitis, a much more serious condition most often seen in adults. The name periodontitis comes from the word *periodontal*, which means "around the tooth," and that is where this serious bacterial infection attacks. In patients afflicted with periodontitis, the gums actually pull away from teeth. Plaque spreads below the gum line, producing toxins that cause irritation and an inflammatory reaction that breaks down tissues and bone around teeth. Eventually this means teeth loosen in the mouth and may have to be removed. Along with tooth decay, periodontal disease is one of the most serious threats to oral health.

Methods for Measuring Gum Disease

Dentists use several methods to examine how far gum disease has spread in a patient's mouth. These tests help determine the best treatment options for a given patient.

- **Gum Probing**: By examining the appearance of your mouth and gums in the office, a dentist can see more clearly how healthy gums are.

- **Signs of inflammation**: Essentially, the dentist will be looking for redness, swelling, and bleeding, as those are beginning signs of gingivitis, the earliest and most reversible form of gum disease.

- **X-rays**: While x-rays don't show gum tissue, they do reveal bone loss around teeth, which is a major warning sign in the area of gum disease.

Causes of Gum Disease

Essentially, gum disease is caused by bacteria. Everyone has bacteria in the mouth, and these bacteria combine with sugar from foods to create plaque—that sticky, harmful substance that adheres to teeth. But although everyone has oral bacteria, a variety of other factors affect what those bacteria are able to do to the gums, from lifestyle choices to genetics.

Genetics

It's undeniable that genetics play a huge role in the way our bodies work, right down to the way the body responds to bacteria. When it comes to gum disease, research shows that about half of the variance in periodontal disease can be linked to genetics.

Dentists see it all the time: there are patients who avoid the dentist for decades and don't practice good oral hygiene yet have no gum disease, and there are other patients who come for regular checkups and meticulously care for their teeth who still battle gum disease.

Q: Can you catch gum disease from someone else?

A: Believe it or not, yes. Research shows, because bacteria that cause gum disease can pass through saliva, it is possible to spread the disease among family members or couples.

Q: Could I be more at risk for gum disease because of my race or ethnicity?

A: As with other infections, gum disease can happen to anyone. However, there are certain races or ethnicities that are more susceptible. African Americans, for example, are especially prone to localized aggressive periodontitis, and both African Americans and Mexican Americans are more likely to deal with periodontal disease than people of European descent.

Certain Habits

Smoking and tobacco are well documented as harmful habits for the lungs, but many people are unaware of how using these substances can also affect the mouth. According to a study published in the *Journal of Periodontology*, smoking is the #1 most influential life habit effecting periodontitis.

Furthermore, another study revealed how secondhand smoke from cigarettes increases risk of bone loss (the leading cause of tooth loss) in patients with periodontitis. Smoking has been shown to be a possible cause for more than half of the cases of adult periodontitis in America.

Medications

Some medications can affect your oral health. Minocycline, which is often prescribed for treatment of acne or rheumatoid arthritis, can cause gum discoloration.

Nifedipine, a drug used to treat high blood pressure, may increase risk for gingival overgrowth, where gums swell and grow over teeth.

These examples demonstrate the importance of giving your dentist a full picture of your medical profile because the drugs you take may change your oral health.

Other Diseases

A variety of other diseases increase a patient's risk for gum disease.

- **Diabetes**: Research shows patients with poorly controlled Type 2 diabetes to be at a higher risk of developing serious periodontal disease.

- **Obesity**: According to a recent study, obesity is a significant predictor of periodontal disease.
  Along the same lines, poor nutrition can weaken the body's immunity and make it more susceptible to infections like periodontal disease.

- **Stress & Depression**: Studies have shown a connection between stress and periodontal diseases. In fact, 57% of studies in one literature review showed a clear link between psychological factors (stress, depression, anxiety, etc.) and gum disease.
  Often, patients with serious depression and/or emotional stress do not take the time to practice good oral hygiene. Research shows, for example, that caregivers older than 50 years of age who take care of relatives with dementia or hypercortisolemia frequently have higher levels of plaque and gingival bleeding.
  Their stressful lifestyle wreaks all kinds of havoc on their bodies, including their mouths. Additionally, hormones can play a role in the health of gums. For women especially, this is a concern, as hormonal changes from puberty, pregnancy, oral contraceptives, or even menopause can affect the mouth.

Links to Other Diseases

Not only can other diseases increase your risk for developing gum disease, but also gum disease can increase your risk for developing other diseases. That's because your body's response to infection in the mouth connects with its response to infection in other places.

Here are a few examples of other diseases linked to gum disease:

Heart Disease

As the leading cause of death in America today, heart disease is a serious matter, the threat of which prompts many of us to go to the gym or to make better dietary choices. Yet beyond diet and exercise, there are other factors that contribute to cardiovascular risk. A recent study shows that patients with periodontal disease have an increased likelihood of developing heart disease.

Therefore, another step to take against heart disease is through the simple tasks of good oral hygiene—such as brushing and flossing regularly—to prevent gum disease from forming or progressing.

Cancer

Research suggests periodontal disease might also increase risk for certain types of cancer for some people. According to one study, men in particular with periodontal disease face a 14% increase of risk in developing cancer compared to men with healthy gums.

Gum Disease Prevention

The best way to prevent gum disease is through good oral hygiene, beginning at a young age—the earlier, the better. By properly caring for your teeth and gums, you fight the damage that bacteria and plaque can cause in your mouth. Just a few minutes of prevention a day can save you from costly and painful consequences later!

Other important steps towards prevention include the following:

- **Physical and Emotional Health** – Taking care of your body reaps many rewards, not least of which is a decreased risk of gum disease. According to one recent study, you do your gums a favor by maintaining a healthy weight and exercising regularly: these activities are not only good for your overall health but also lower your chances of periodontal disease.

- **Regular Dental Visits** – Along with regularly flossing and brushing your teeth, an important part of good oral hygiene is regular dental visits. Your dentist will be able to probe gums, look for early signs of inflammation, and perform x-rays to measure bone loss.

- **Awareness of Family History** – Because genetics play such a big role in periodontal disease, if you have siblings with gum disease or if your parents lost their teeth or suffered from gum disease at a young age, you need to be especially vigilant.

- **Vitamins** – Good nutritional intake of vitamins such as C and D can help prevent periodontal disease. Calcium also, according to one recent study, is an important and beneficial nutrient: a low intake of calcium results in more serious gum disease.

Treatment

Time and research have shown there's no magic pill or wonder drug to treat gum disease. Because it stems from bacteria residing in plaque and calculus, we need to manually remove the plaque and calculus (tartar) in order to remove the damage. Lasers are increasingly being used to aid in removal of bacteria and plaque from the mouth. Additionally, medicinal rinses and antibiotics can aid in controlling the level of bacteria in the mouth.

Depending on the severity, treatment for gum disease can be non-surgical or surgical. In non-surgical treatment, the teeth are thoroughly cleaned beneath the gum-line. The goal here is to reduce the plaque and bacteria and allow for proper healing. Lasers can be used to aid in disinfecting the gum pockets, and antibiotics or disinfectants can be placed beneath the gum line. Using modern technology, many patients avoid the more invasive gum surgery. In traditional gum surgery, the gums are separated from the teeth with a scalpel and the roots are cleaned. Stitches are used to place the gums back in place. Unfortunately, this invasive method is still being used by many dentists to treat patients that would respond well to non-surgical laser treatment. In our opinion, traditional gum surgery should be reserved ONLY for extremely severe cases or where non-surgical methods have not been successful.

Laser Treatment

Laser treatments offer a modern, gentler alternative in treating gum disease. Unlike the invasive and uncomfortable option of surgery, lasers cause less bleeding, swelling, and pain; plus, when combined with scaling and root planning, laser treatments can be very effective.

One exciting laser option is Deep Pocket Therapy (DPT) with New Attachment™ using the Waterlase MD™ laser and Radial Firing Perio Tip™. Minimally invasive and cleared by the FDA, this therapy treats moderate to advanced periodontitis. It's especially effective at removing subgingival inflamed tissue and calculus, preparing those areas for healing and new attachment.

Research shows that the Er,Cr:YSSG laser energy of the Waterlase® MD in particular provides exciting new treatment options for restorative dentistry and surgical procedures. In a recent study, 49 pediatric patients underwent restorative procedures or oral surgery done with an Er,Cr:YSSG laser, and none of them needed local anesthesia. Yet reducing pain levels is obviously not only beneficial for pediatric dental patients but also adults. Contrasted with surgery, laser treatments offer a much more comfortable experience.

Bernard's Story

When Bernard remembers going to the dentist as a child, he remembers the smell of Novocain and the sound of a drill, both of which still make him nervous today. The first oral surgery he had was the traditional "scalpel" kind—painful and scary, leaving him nervous about the dentist even later in life. That's why he was so surprised by his recent experience with laser treatment: It was a total contrast. He hardly felt any pain at all!

New Developments

The hot topic in periodontology today is inflammation. Linked with all kinds of diseases, from Alzheimer's to diabetes, inflammation is also associated with gum disease, which is essentially chronic inflammation caused by oral bacteria. Periodontal disease increases inflammation in the body, elevating the C-reactive protein, which in turn increases risk for other health conditions as serious as heart disease.

Gum Disease & Inflammation

The connection between gum disease and inflammation is an important one. It means that blood markers of inflammation such as C-reactive protein can be used as markers for gum disease. It also means treating gum disease to reduce the C-reactive protein may indirectly treat other inflammation-based conditions.

Dentures

What Are Dentures?

Dentures are essentially removable false teeth, available in two forms: full or partial. Full dentures replace an entire set of upper or lower teeth, and partial dentures replace one or a certain number of teeth. While this area of dentistry has seen many improvements over the last few years, dentures can still feel strange to patients, especially in the beginning. Dentures require adjustments and regular maintenance, and they can affect a patient's eating, speaking, and sensitivity to temperatures of food and liquids. According to a recent study evaluating the effect of removable partial dentures on periodontal health, the design of the dentures can also affect the health of the mouth; because partial dentures can increase the risk for gum disease, a good fit and careful oral hygiene are essential in protecting against gum disease and other dental problems.

What often makes dentures most difficult is the psychological effect they have on patients. Putting teeth in and out of your mouth on a regular basis can be very hard emotionally: you're regularly reminded of something abnormal and uncomfortable about yourself. Because of their reputation and history, dentures can also make patients feel old, which is very discouraging and hard to deal with. Plus, dentures are by nature bulky inside the mouth. This is true of even the best dentures, and it's common for them to cause limitations on what you can eat; however, there can be some improvement with denture adhesive.

Dentures Lead to Bone Resorption

Another problem with dentures is that when they are worn over time, the bone resorbs. This happens because healthy teeth are secured in the jawbone, so when a tooth is lost, the bone doesn't need to be there anymore, and it will gradually resorb or shrink.

Over the years, the dentures need to be made thicker to compensate for the loss, and the more time that goes by, the thicker and thicker the dentures need to be made. Dentures constantly need adjustment.

With dentures, patients are continually losing bone because there is no use for the bone. Dentures are secured with bad-tasting glue that can actually cause a gagging sensation. Implants, on the other hand, mimic the structure of natural teeth and are secured right in the bone. Therefore, implants actually stop the bone from resorbing and definitely help preserve the bone you do have, allowing you to have a younger looking smile.

Dump Your Dentures for Good with Implants

We recommend implants, as opposed to dentures, because they are permanently embedded in the bone, just like natural teeth, so they do not come out like dentures. They are very natural, healthy, stable, and functional; plus, they preserve your bone. They are a permanent, low-maintenance solution.

While dentures require continual maintenance, implants only need regular professional cleanings and daily brushing and flossing. Patients care for them just like natural teeth, and with proper maintenance, they can last forever.

When a patient can eliminate floppy dentures, it means being able to taste foods again, and getting to experience a whole new world of flavors. Think about it: no more yucky-tasting denture glue. No more anxiety over feeling old because of ill-fitting dentures. A free and clear palate to enjoy tastes freely.

By getting rid of dentures, patients take back their lives: no more choosing from a menu of soft foods that can be eaten without embarrassment, but instead a whole wide world of delicious tastes and textures waiting to be explored and rediscovered. All of these benefits are possible with cutting-edge technology and skilled dental specialists.

Implants

When it comes to replacing missing teeth, implants are, in most cases, the best option because they preserve the tooth structure of adjacent teeth. Implants don't need to be connected to other teeth and can't decay, making them an especially effective, permanent option for people who have had severe caries/decay in the past.

Implants are small titanium screws that are placed under the gum and allow real, secure, prosthetic teeth to be inserted in the place of natural teeth. Because implants get fused directly to your jawbone, they are able to give valuable stability to artificial teeth, bridges, or dentures, keeping them from sliding around in your mouth. That secure fit is what creates the more natural feel that implants promise. Implants can be used to replace one or more teeth without affecting intact adjacent teeth, or they can provide support and security for a bridge or a denture.

The process may sound painful, especially for someone who has dental fear, but it can be literally painless. The biggest factors that affect the experience are the complexity of the case and the skill of the dentist. In many cases, patients will not need a single painkiller after implants are placed by a skilled dentist.

Implants have become more popular in the last twenty years, and are widely recommended because of their history. Time-tested, implants can last a very long time, ultimately forever. They're easy, quick, and painless when done properly. The only caveat is that implants must be done precisely and accurately. Again, this is why patients should only trust a dental specialist, such as a periodontist or an oral surgeon to surgically place implants.

Thanks to continued progress in new technologies, modern-day dental implants have become the preferred treatment option for millions of people today. The truth is dental implants can make an enormous difference in the life of a patient, ending the all-too-common embarrassment and frustration associated with missing teeth or ill-fitting dentures.

Through innovative dental specialists, there are new and proven technologies available that offer clients ingenious, personalized solutions to their dental challenges. Unlike status quo dentists, experienced dental specialists offer patients new options and have them walking out of their office with a new smile—in just a few comfortable visits.

The Implant Process

During the implant procedure, patients are numb and comfortable, and certainly if sedation is involved, there will be an even greater level of comfort. Sedated patients can rest in twilight while their work is done and then wake up with no recollection of the process.

With sedation, patients feel like their implants were placed in minutes, and all dental fears and anxieties melt away. Even if no sedation is involved, it is possible for patients to be expertly numb and comfortable. Sedation is a patient's choice. Post-operatively, a mild painkiller is prescribed; but in most cases, patients will come back for a follow-up appointment and admit they never needed a single pill.

Implants can be stronger than real teeth, certainly stronger than dentures. Implants do not bend, and they don't come out. They are permanent. Everything is connected and secured.

People who have some missing teeth and some original teeth that are still healthy should also consider implants, as implants would benefit a patient who doesn't have back teeth but still has front teeth that are in decent condition. Although that person might feel the back teeth are not important, the truth is that restoration is vital. When back teeth are missing, the front teeth will eventually decline due to the increased pressure placed on them.

When the pressure of eating and other oral functions are not distributed evenly between the front and back teeth, the teeth carrying the entire burden will eventually decline. On the other hand, if implants with crowns are inserted to replace missing back teeth, a patient can preserve the natural front teeth and have a natural, functional, and beautiful smile.

Availability of Implants

Over the last 30 years, there have been significant advances in the dental field. Usually when a tooth cannot be saved, it is removed. Sometimes this leaves a hole, and other times, depending on the number of teeth lost, bridges or dentures are necessary. Implants, which have been available for a while, are unfortunately not usually offered by many dentists. There are a couple reasons for this.

First, insurance companies discourage them because they do not want to cover them. This is a shame because implants are a much more natural, functional, and healthy solution than other tooth replacement options. But insurance companies do affect the options presented to patients. Another issue is that most dentists will wait several months after placing an implant before inserting a permanent tooth. This is not ideal for the patient or the dentist.

The truth is that implants are superior to traditional bridges and dentures, both of which present serious health issues and are difficult to keep clean. In fact, recent research shows that bridges can no longer be called the standard of care for restoration of a missing tooth.

Through new technologies that measure implant stability and healing progress, patients return home immediately after treatment with nice-looking smiles and no missing teeth. Implants can be placed right away, and in the right situation and the right circumstance, the final crown can be placed within weeks. Thanks to new technologies, dentists can move the restoration process along quickly, which is good news for patients who want quicker results and are willing to push the envelope utilizing the unique technology and experience of specialists.

Ellie's Story

As a lawyer, Ellie deals with people face-to-face every single day, so taking care of her appearance has been a really important priority not just for her personal life, but also for her career. For as long as she can remember, the one area of her looks that she was never fully comfortable about was her teeth—until last year when she got implants. By replacing some of her missing teeth with complete implants, she finally has the smile she always wanted, not to mention the confidence. Ellie described the process as "painless and perfectly orchestrated." In her case, a 3-D CT scan was utilized to properly plan for the implant placement. With her busy schedule, Ellie didn't want to be sent to a radiology center where she would have to make an appointment and wait to be seen. However, Ellie was fortunate to have chosen a dentist with the 3-D scanner on premises, so getting the scan didn't disrupt her schedule or cost her more financially. After the scan, Ellie was scheduled for the implant placement. During the procedure, Ellie was comfortably sedated and four implants were placed along with beautiful temporary crowns. Ellie's healing was uneventful and completely painless. When Ellie returned for a follow-up visit, she said that she didn't even need a single pain pill and that she was immediately able to enjoy her food in ways that she hasn't enjoyed it in a decade. Four weeks later, permanent porcelain crowns were inserted and Ellie continues to enjoy her new teeth. "My only regret is that I wish I had done it sooner," she says.

Neil's Story

Many clients are embarrassed when they first seek dental help. Neil was a good example. A very nice-looking man who dressed well, Neil had a long moustache and didn't smile often. When he first came into his dental office, he was afraid to open his mouth and reveal the depth of his tooth problems. He told the dentist, "I'm very embarrassed. You've never seen a mouth as bad as mine." What he didn't realize is that specialists have seen it all. An x-ray revealed Neil only had two or three roots left in his upper gums; he had a malfunctioning denture. Up until that point, he'd kept the denture inside his mouth with glue in order to avoid seeing a dentist; but by seeking treatment, he found a life-changing solution that included implants.

After taking detailed measurements beforehand, the dentist scheduled Neil's treatment. On the day of the procedure, he was sedated; three hours later, he woke up to a perfect, natural-looking smile that he was proud to show off. He threw away his dentures and has never looked back.

What Makes Implants Work?

Thanks to research and discoveries made in recent years, today's modern dental implants are able to combat the previous problems associated with replacing teeth. By using the right materials and methods, dentists are able to effectively implant artificial teeth in a way that the body accepts well and responds to.

The Right Methods

Today, dentists take important measures to make implants as effective as possible. First, they must be fastidious about contamination, not allowing anything unnecessary to touch the surgical site and cause infection. In order to avoid any injury to the bone in surgery, they use special tools and drills to both prepare the bone and to prevent the buildup of heat from interfering with healing.

Osteogenesis and Osseointegration

After placing an implant, a dentist usually allows the implant to "rest" beneath the gum for a period of time, so that healing can be complete. The process in which your body develops new bone cells up and around the implant is called osteogenesis, and the overall healing process, acceptance, and stability creation for implants is called osseointegration. Once the implant has fully integrated into your mouth, it offers strong support for artificial teeth.

Q: Is there a chance my body will reject my implant?

A: Although implants can fail, the chance is very rare. Because the titanium that implants are made from is a totally biocompatible material, your body should accept an implant as easily as natural tissues and teeth.

Timing of Implants

Traditionally speaking, implants are a multi-step process, requiring surgery, healing time, and then restoration. While the exact timing is different for each individual, the entire process typically takes 2-4 months to be fully completed.

Placement to Restoration

During implant surgery, the dentist inserts small titanium posts below the gum line. A temporary tooth can be placed on the implant immediately or at a later time after osseointegration is complete – usually in 2-4 months.

Regardless of whether a temporary tooth was placed onto the implant immediately or not, a permanent tooth will usually be made after the osseointegration period of 2-4 months. The new permanent teeth will be fitted and adjusted for just the right size, shape, color, and fit. After restoration is complete, you'll have functional, aesthetically pleasing teeth, just like the originals.

Time Between Placement & New Tooth

As mentioned above, after a new implant has been placed, there is usually a period of healing before a new permanent tooth can be added. Fortunately, there are a variety of steps that can minimize the waiting time and make it less uncomfortable for patients.

Immediate Temporization
vs. Removable Temporary

Immediate temporization is the term used to describe inserting a temporary tooth directly on an implant immediately. Although removable temporary teeth (i.e., flippers) are another option, experienced implant dentists and their patients dislike them. Beyond just the undesirable aesthetics, removable teeth are psychologically difficult. Nobody wants that constant inconvenience and reminder of what is missing.

"Immediate Load" and Early Load Implants

Certain patients may be eligible for early or immediately loaded implants rather than the traditional longer process. Increasingly popular, these alternatives have one thing in common: they lessen the overall treatment time and completely eliminate the use of a temporary denture. Immediate or early implant loading provides excellent aesthetic and functional results, as well as good experiences for patients due to its quickness.

"Immediate Load" Implants

Immediately loaded implants allow patients to have new teeth installed on the implants on the same day as the surgery. Their benefits are numerous: shorter overall treatment and surgery times, better gum aesthetics, secure fixed prostheses, and better patient satisfaction.

Research has shown that immediate loading decreases treatment time and patient discomfort. Also, according to a recent study of 979 patients in a two-year period, immediately loaded implants give predictable success—99.4% in the anterior and 97% in the posterior mandible in that study.

Many factors go into the decision of when to load an implant with a temporary or permanent tooth. A good and experienced implant dentist can help you decide which course of treatment is right for you.

Early Load Implants

Early loading involves placing the temporary or final tooth restoration soon after surgery, usually within a few weeks. According to a recent study, early loading is a better option than delayed loading (2-6 months after surgery) for patients, as delay in loading implants seems to increase marginal bone loss.

Osstell® Technology

Many studies have been conducted to evaluate the effectiveness of immediate and early loading of implants. An important tool in that analysis is the Osstell® resonance frequency analyzer (RFA). Osstell® offers a non-invasive technology used to determine an implant's stability at two different stages: at placement, and before loading. Technological advances in implant dentistry, such as Osstell®, allow the whole process to be done more quickly and effectively.

Whatever the timing of your implant, the most important outcome is that after restoration, the implant looks and feels like a natural part of your mouth.

The Truth about Implant Specialists

As in any field of modern medicine, dentistry has several types of specialists who focus on particular aspects of teeth, be they pediatric dentists that specialize in children's dentistry or periodontists who focus on gum disease. Yet not all specializations are alike. Some professionals may claim to be implant specialists, for example, but the truth is that there is no such recognized designation. While oral surgeons, periodontists, and prosthodontists all receive advanced training for their division of specialty, so-called implant specialists do not.

Therefore, it's a better option to find a qualified specialist (such as a prosthodontist or periodontist) who has the experience, knowledge, and skill to work with implants—and you should do your homework to find an excellent implant specialist because serious complications can occur from implant surgery.

What to Look for in an Implant Dentist

You should ask questions of your implant dentist as if he were applying for a position at a company you own. By knowing how to ask the right questions of your dentist, you'll know how to determine what level of skill and knowledge he or she offers in the area of implants. This way, you'll have the comfort and peace of mind of knowing you're working with an experienced professional.

Some questions to ask your dentist include:

- What implant experience do you have?
- How often do you place implants?
- Are you a general dentist or a specialist?
- What type of training have you had in the area of implants?

Perfecting Implant Restorations

Not all implants, or the dentists who place them, are

created equal. In reality, it takes specialized care, skill, and experience to make implant restorations look perfect. Sometimes, in dentistry as in the rest of life, the old adage, "You get what you pay for," is really true.

Dentists who stay on the cutting-edge of implant developments will know about key technologies and changes affecting the field. An awareness of new features like zirconia abutment posts and crowns, as well as knowledge of tissue sculpting, can make the difference between an average result and a superb one.

Overdentures

The conventional dentures of the past were uncomfortable, loose fitting, and bothersome. For some patients, dentures also affected the way they could talk and eat, acting as a constant reminder that their teeth were no longer normal.

Today, there are better options. For those patients who cannot afford full implant-supported teeth, implant *overdentures* are an excellent, less expensive alternative to traditional dentures. In *overdentures*, implants are used to attach to and secure removable dentures to aid in stabilization and fit, improving patient satisfaction significantly as compared to traditional dentures. One study showed specifically in elderly patients that wearing implant *overdentures* made a positive difference in nutrition and overall quality of life.

Another study further proved high overall patient satisfaction with *overdentures*—regardless of age, gender, length of follow-up, and several other factors. What's more, *overdentures* have been proven to improve maximum bite force and masticatory performance even over a 10-year period. In addition to the personal benefits that *overdentures* offer patients, they also are cost-efficient. While not as effective as non-removable restorations, they are considerably lower in cost.

New Technologies

Exciting new developments in the field of implants offer potential for even better quality treatment and patient satisfaction. Two especially promising new technologies are zirconia implants and computer-guided surgeries.

Zirconia Implants

Up until recently, titanium and titanium alloys have been the material of choice for implants, but zirconia implants offer a suitable alternative in terms of color, properties, and biocompatibility. A recent study has shown that zirconia implants provide comparable osseointegration to titanium, making them an acceptable implant substance. Although only available in very limited supply in the United States, zirconia implants have been promoted as a possible substitute to titanium for more than a decade. Zirconia bioceramic offers many benefits, such as improved biocompatibility and low radioactivity.

Computer-Guided Surgery

Another new technology growing in popularity in the field of dental implants is computer-guided surgery. Utilizing CT-Scan data and a thorough pre-operative assessment, dentists are able to plan the implant placement prior to the surgery. A computer-designed drill guide is made and directs the dentist to the exact location of the planned implant. This allows the restoration tooth to be made with ideal dimensions and aesthetic appearance.

Full Mouth Restoration
A Healthy, Functional, and Beautiful Smile

One of the last things you want as a dental patient is to lose teeth without a careful plan of their replacement. Pulling teeth out should be an absolute last resort for dentists, and when it does have to happen, it should be done precisely the right way.

The good news is that no matter how many teeth a person is missing, or if the condition of the existing teeth are poor, a beautiful smile is still possible, and along with it comes a sense of youth, beauty, and confidence. *Full Mouth Restoration* may include implants, root canals, extractions or crowns, depending upon each patient's unique needs and conditions. All necessary procedures can be performed with virtually no pain, in a few hours, while you rest in peaceful twilight.

Missing Teeth and Eating

Missing or severely broken teeth significantly impact a person's ability to enjoy food, entertainment, and gatherings with friends and family. Eating is involved in so many parts of life and is what sustains life, not to mention offering growth, enjoyment, entertainment, social interaction, and a sense of community.

Because eating plays such a key role in most social events, from holiday gatherings, dates, and weddings to job interviews and business functions, missing and broken teeth can dramatically affect a person's quality of life.

Think about it: when you are missing teeth, it's easier for food particles to get stuck in empty crevices or adjacent teeth, creating embarrassing situations or, in some cases, even choking hazards. Living with missing teeth isn't just less attractive than a healthy smile; it's a problem that leads to all kinds of uncomfortable situations. Many clients with missing teeth have low confidence in eating situations. Because eating is so closely intertwined with business, relationships, and family events, it really can negatively impact one's life.

Thankfully though, you don't have to settle for a life with missing teeth. There is a clear solution to your unique set of dental challenges. Even if you already have dentures or bridges, there are new ideas to explore. Whatever your situation, you don't have to miss out on life.

Tooth Removal Is Not the Only Option

Gum disease is the number one reason for tooth loss in our country. While it starts out as a quiet and painless problem, it slowly grows and extends through the mouth until it reaches a point where a tooth starts hurting. By the time the pain begins the disease will have spread far enough to loosen teeth, and there may be nothing a dentist can do to save them.

It is possible to detect and treat gum disease easily through regular dental visits on at least a biannual basis. The problem is that so many people avoid dentists because of fear and anxiety that they never catch the disease in its early stages. Many people think that if nothing hurts, everything must be fine—but with initially painless gum disease, that is not the case.

Intraoral bacteria are seeping down into the gums, wreaking havoc, eating away the gum and the bone that support the teeth. As the disease progresses, the teeth start getting looser and looser, the spaces between teeth enlarge, affecting a person's general health and appearance.

The goal should always be to save your teeth. If there is a good possibility of saving the tooth, that is what should be done, whether that means utilizing the latest in laser technology for gum treatment or using more extensive procedures. The benefit of laser gum treatment is that it is wonderfully less invasive than a scalpel and stitches. It works nicely to totally kill the bacteria causing the disease. Sometimes though, a tooth needs to be saved with a root canal, where there are salvageable teeth that have a lot of cavities, decay, or breaks.

Would You Rather See a Generalist Or a Specialist?

The difference between a generalist and specialist is training. A general dentist gets his or her degree from a dental school. As a rule, general dentists offer a scope of procedures, from minor fillings to simple root canals.

In today's world of dentistry, there have been so many advances that no dentist can competently perform *all* available procedures. That is why there are specialists who choose particular areas of dentistry to master. While an experienced general dentist can provide quality treatment, he or she is typically a jack-of-all-trades, master of none. Specialists are the masters—but only of one or two highly specialized procedures.

A dental specialist chooses a particular area of expertise, such as periodontics, prosthodontics, endodontics, or orthodontics. Then, after completing dental school, the dentist completes additional selective processes to be accepted into the chosen specialty.

Every specialist undergoes two to three years of additional training to master the specialty work: this is full-time training that involves working with actual patients. That way, when a specialist is done with training, he or she not only has academic but also experiential knowledge. That is how specialists master certain areas of dentistry: they hone their skills in real-world situations with real patients. Their experience doesn't come only from the theoretical but also from the practical, working in the trenches with patients who have real problems and real fears. Each specialist is a master of something different.

When you see a team of specialists, you can be more comfortable with the plan to restore your teeth, knowing that treatments are done appropriately and expertly, with an overall concept of what will work best to restore your teeth, oral health, and confidence.

Specialists can treat any case in their chosen field, regardless of age, background, or dental condition, because all the different patients have certain commonalities. That is why specialists are the best resource for transforming your smile no matter what condition your mouth is in, and they know how to give you back your smile, youth, and confidence.

Maintaining A New Smile

A new smile is like a jumpstart on life, something that turns back the hands of time and gives you a chance to start over—and practicing good oral hygiene is one of the best ways to take care of that fresh start. After phobic patients conquer their fears through IV sedation and are able to receive treatment, it makes sense to want to protect that investment, as well as avoid the need to go through it all again. The key is good oral hygiene.

Just like a morning shower invigorates and refreshes your body, so daily brushing and flossing your teeth makes you feel rejuvenated and healthy. By keeping your teeth and gums clean, you protect yourself from sickness, prevent growth of bacteria, fight infections, and even lift your emotional spirits. The importance of good oral hygiene cannot be overstated. It's the best way to care for your teeth and gums, as well as to prevent future oral problems.

Prevention of Cavities

The single best prevention against cavities is good oral hygiene. By regularly cleansing and caring for your teeth, you protect them from the build-up of plaque and tartar that can lead to tooth decay. In fact, the oral hygiene practiced in today's society, both at home and through regular dental visits, explains the biggest improvements in oral diseases to date. Yet oral hygiene isn't only important for prevention of cavities; it also yields other important benefits.

Pleasant Breath

One of the most obvious benefits of practicing good oral hygiene is pleasant breath. Bad breath results from bacteria growing in your mouth, particularly in the crevices between teeth, where it releases sulfur compounds that create a bad smell. By cleansing your teeth and gums regularly, you keep that bacteria at bay and keep your breath smelling fresh.

Prevention of Gum Disease & Gingivitis

Good oral hygiene not only protects your teeth against cavities, but it also prevents the serious inflammation of gum disease and gingivitis. Most adults in America have some form of gum disease, ranging from mild inflammation to severe bone damage. Gum disease, which is created by long-term plaque deposits left unchecked can be prevented simply through proper oral hygiene. By removing sticky plaque before it's able to harden into tartar and inflame gums, the disease is stopped before it can progress, protecting your mouth from serious damage.

Q: Will chewing gum affect the health of my teeth and gums?

A: Yes! Actually, you may be surprised to know the positive impact chewing gum may have on your mouth. A recent study has shown that chewing a sugar free gum stimulates flow of saliva, which helps cleanse food and plaque from teeth and therefore decreases risk for gingivitis, periodontitis, and decay.

Types of Toothpaste

Good oral hygiene begins with brushing your teeth. By keeping up with this important habit, you cleanse your teeth of harmful bacteria and help prevent oral disease. Part of this cleansing routine involves toothpaste.

Usually, toothpaste contains a combination of four types of ingredients: abrasives to remove bacteria and stains, humectants to prevent water loss, thickeners that make the toothpaste hold together, and flavorings that make it taste better.

When choosing a type of toothpaste, you have many variations to consider. While for the most part toothpastes are the same, several have been made that cater to specific needs and problems. Certain varieties will also have extra ingredients for specific needs.

Here are a few varieties of specialty toothpastes available:

- **Desensitizing:** For people with sensitive teeth, a desensitizing toothpaste (such as Sensodyne® or Arm & Hammer® Advance White® for Sensitive Teeth) can be helpful, as it has an ingredient called Potassium Nitrate, designed specifically to help oral sensitivity.

- **Extra Fluoride**: For people with a high rate of cavities, there are toothpastes (such as Prevident® 5000+) designed with extra fluoride to help remineralization of the teeth; however, these high-fluoride toothpastes are only available by prescription. Also, if you use any fluoride products, be careful not to swallow it: too much fluoride can be harmful.

- **Whitening**: Many people today are concerned about discoloration of teeth, and so whitening toothpastes offer a cleansing routine that may somewhat brighten enamel. The key ingredient in a whitening toothpaste is an abrasive, made to remove existing teeth stains and prevent future teeth stains without harming oral tissues.

Q: Which toothpaste is best?

A: Generally speaking, all toothpastes are the same. However, the type that's best for you may depend on your individual needs, which is why it's helpful to consider all varieties available. We recommend Colgate® Total® and, for sensitive teeth, Sensodyne® Pronamel® Toothpaste for Sensitive Teeth.

Fluoride

Because of its power in preventing and fighting tooth decay, fluoride is an important part of good oral hygiene. Its benefits are so far reaching, the U.S. Surgeon General has called community water fluoridation the most economical and safe way to protect people from tooth decay. That's why fluoride is such a popular ingredient in toothpaste today.

Benefits of Fluoride

According to the Centers for Disease Control and Prevention, brushing twice daily with fluoride toothpaste is one of the easiest ways to keep decay from occurring.

This ingredient strengthens enamel, reverses the decay process, and is easily available. For people with weakened enamel or existing decay, this is excellent news, as fluoride offers not just prevention but also treatment of damage.

Dangers of Too Much Fluoride

Despite its many benefits, fluoride can be dangerous in large doses. Swallowing an excessive amount of fluoridated toothpaste can be very harmful and may cause various symptoms including stomach pain, diarrhea, and other serious problems.

For this reason, fluoride should be used thoughtfully, without swallowing. Then, as long as you're brushing twice daily, you will reap all the benefits of this beneficial nutrient.

Non-Fluoride Toothpastes

If you're concerned about the harmful effects of fluoride, there are several non-fluoride varieties available. Remember though that eliminating fluoride means eliminating its benefits, including prevention of tooth decay. Non-fluoride toothpaste is best for patients who are not prone to dental decay or have dental implants replacing all their teeth (since implants don't decay).

Sensitive Teeth

As anyone with sensitive teeth can tell you, when teeth

are worn down, some of the simplest pleasures—eating a bowl of ice cream, drinking hot coffee—can become painful and frustrating. One of the most common complaints among dental patients, sensitive teeth are not only uncomfortable, but they are also more susceptible to decay.

Causes of Sensitive Teeth

The outer layer of your teeth is the hardest substance in your whole body, protecting the crown; below that, something called cementum protects roots under the gum line. Beneath these two substances is dentin, a less dense part of the tooth with lots of small hollow areas where hot, cold, and very sweet foods are able to get in and stimulate nerves.

What happens with sensitive teeth is that when the enamel wears down, as a result of certain habits and diet choices, the dentin is exposed. This means heightened sensations in response to hot and cold drinks or food, as well as increased susceptibility to cavities.

Gum recession also contributes to teeth sensitivity. In this condition, lost gum tissue leaves the roots of teeth exposed. This too can cause sensitivity, as the exposure makes it easier for food and bacteria to reach nerves.

Treatment for Sensitive Teeth

One of the most important ways to treat sensitive teeth is through proper oral hygiene. For people with sensitive teeth, in addition to brushing twice daily and flossing daily, it's wise to use a soft-bristled toothbrush and to choose a toothpaste suitable for your needs. Toothpaste for sensitive teeth has ingredients that clog the little canals in teeth, protecting your nerves from irritation.

When sensitivity persists for more than three days, you should see your dentist. In cases of decay or cracks, you may need a filling or crown to protect from further damage. There's also something called a desensitizing agent that your dentist can apply to sensitive teeth, which can help prevent nerve irritation.

Q: How can I avoid tooth sensitivity?

A: Know what lifestyle choices increase the risk of sensitivity, such as high consumption of acidic foods like citrus juices and soft drinks, conditions such as bulimia and acid reflux disease, and poor oral hygiene.

Q: How long will it take for a specialty toothpaste to
provide relief?

A: In most cases, you'll need to regularly use a toothpaste made for sensitive teeth for at least a month before noticing any major changes.

Toothbrushes: Manual or Electric?

For good oral hygiene, the American Dental Association recommends brushing your teeth twice daily.

Generally speaking, we find electric toothbrushes to be most effective for patients; however, patients with excellent oral hygiene who have successfully used manual brushes should keep doing so. The saying really is as true with teeth as it is with everything else: it's not so much the tool, but *how you use it*!

Manual Toothbrushes

There are two primary types of manual toothbrushes: soft-bristled and hard-bristled. Avoid using hard-bristled toothbrushes, as they can be too harsh on your gums. The truth is, you don't need hard bristles or intense pressure to clean your teeth. It's better to use a soft-bristled brush and to glide it across your teeth in a gentle manner.

Electric Toothbrushes

Many patients find electric toothbrushes more enjoyable to use. According to the Academy of General Dentistry, these brushes have been able to motivate reluctant brushers to clean their teeth, making them a great invention indeed.

Plus, electric toothbrushes aren't just fun; we also find people can be more effective with them. In a recent study, dental professionals saw positive change in 80.5% of patients who used an electric toothbrush, including better gum condition and removal of plaque.

Flossing

When it comes to oral hygiene, no habit is harder to take on than flossing—even for dentists! Nonetheless, flossing is definitely worth the effort, as it yields unparalleled benefits. Nothing else can get in between the teeth, right into those hidden nooks where cavities form, the way floss can. In fact, the American Dental Association advises flossing every day in order to most effectively remove plaque and food particles stuck between teeth and under gums.

Types of Floss
- Woven: Gentle on gums
- Waxed: Slick for sliding easily between tight teeth
- Teflon: Made especially for tight spaces
- Wide: Ideal if you have a lot of bridgework

Today's market also offers a variety of alternative flossing methods, from picks and sticks to brushes. Some of these wonderful new products make flossing less annoying and much more enjoyable.

Floss Threaders

A floss threader is a pointed plastic loop designed to get floss into hard-to-reach places like beneath bridges or between braces. This tool can guide floss through tricky spots to ensure removal of plaque.

Other Flossing Aids

For people who have a difficult time working floss between teeth, there are many flossing aids available. From brushes to picks and disposable picks you can use and throw away, you'll find there might be an option that makes the task easier for you. These aids often have slim handles that make them easier to control than traditional floss thread.

Waterpik®

One of the best flossing tools on the market today is the Waterpik®. Even for us, it makes the process of flossing so much easier and fun! The Waterpik® is also called a water flosser, a dental water jet, or an oral irrigator. It was designed specifically to improve gum health, and it has been proven to be more effective than regular floss. According to one study, the Waterpik® is actually 93% more effective than string floss at reducing gingival bleeding.

There is a bit of a learning curve in using the Waterpik®: the first time you try it out, you might feel like a hurricane went through your bathroom, leaving water everywhere! But once you get the hang of it, you may find it a preferable flossing option.

That said, as much as we like the Waterpik®, it isn't for everyone. For patients with extensive plaque and tartar below the gum line, it can push that damage even deeper under the gums. For that reason, we recommend seeing a dentist for a periodontal evaluation and a thorough cleansing before using a Waterpik®.

Fresh Breath

Bad breath is no laughing matter, especially to those you suffer from it. In most cases, bacteria are to blame, although sometimes more serious gastric and sinus problems are the root. Whatever the case, all the habits of good oral hygiene encourage fresh breath, from regular brushing to daily flossing. That's because a clean mouth smells better, and by keeping your mouth clean, you improve your breath!

- **Brush your tongue:** When brushing your teeth, take time to also gently brush your tongue. Your tongue harbors lots of germs that can create bad breath.

- **Watch what you eat:** Certain foods may temporarily cause unpleasant breath as they affect your mouth, transfer to bloodstream and lungs, and get expelled through your mouth. To see if your diet is causing problems for your breath, log what you eat and track the changes.

- **See your dentist if bad breath continues:** It's not just poor oral hygiene that causes bad breath. See your dentist if you have dry mouth (xerostomia), which decreases saliva, results from certain medications or conditions, and makes breath smell.

  Tobacco products may also lead to bad breath, among other oral problems, and your dentist may be able to help you stop the habit. Your dentist will also be able to tell you if the breath problem stems from something other than your mouth, in which case you may want to see a general physician. These causes may include infections, postnasal drip, gastrointestinal illness, diabetes, or liver or kidney problems.

Q: Is oral hygiene still important if my bad breath comes from another source?

A: Yes! No matter the cause of bad breath, you will benefit from good oral hygiene.

Mouth Rinses

According to the American Dental Association, antimicrobial mouth rinses reduce bacteria and their activity in plaque, which means they essentially work against gingivitis. Convenient and inexpensive, mouth rinses take very little time to implement in your regular routine.

Mouth rinses usually contain a blend of basic ingredients such as water, cleansers, flavors, colorings, and sometimes alcohol, which can potentially dry out the mouth. These components combine with active ingredients like fluoride, astringent salts, or antimicrobial agents that help reduce plaque.

Fluoride mouth rinses: Available over the counter, these products have a small percentage of sodium fluoride, which attacks plaque in your mouth. Higher strength rinses are available by prescription only.

Antiseptic mouth rinses: Antimicrobial agents combat the bacteria in your mouth to prevent oral disease and bad breath.

The Natural Dentist® Mouth Rinse: We recommend The Natural Dentist® mouth rinse, both because it is effective and because it is made with all natural, safe ingredients. A recent study has shown The Natural Dentist® Healthy Gums Oral Rinse to work better than Listerine® at limiting the growth of bacteria in the mouth. Created from herbal extracts, it helps treat even serious gum issues.

Whatever kind you choose, remember a mouth rinse does not substitute for brushing and flossing, but rather it is an extra weapon in the fight against plaque and build up of germs.

Q: Do all mouth rinses help reduce plaque?
A: No. Cosmetic mouth rinses only deodorize and freshen the mouth, providing a temporary solution for bad breath. Only mouth rinses with active ingredients made to combat bacteria will help reduce plaque.

Q: Should I brush first or rinse first?
A: According to the American Dental Association, whether you brush, floss, or rinse first, it makes no difference.

Brushing Techniques

When it comes to brushing your teeth, method is key. The way you take care of them can make all the difference—not just in preventing cavities but in keeping your teeth for a lifetime!

Here are a few tips to keep in mind:

- **Begin brushing early:** There's a reason we're always telling kids to brush their teeth: good oral hygiene begins at a young age! The sooner you start caring for your teeth, the greater the rewards.

- **Take your time:** If you're only spending a minute or so brushing your teeth each morning, you're not brushing long enough. Although most of the population spends only around 45 seconds brushing, a recent study has shown that patients need to brush for at least two minutes to really remove plaque and reap noticeable benefits.

- **Don't press too hard:** Using too much pressure with your toothbrush can lead to gum recession and tooth abrasion. Remember, the technique is more important than the tool! Be gentle with your brush, and work slowly.

- **Be thorough:** Good brushing begins with the outer sides of your teeth, moves to the inner teeth, and continues to the flat chewing surfaces. Place your brush at a 45-degree angle and gently move it back and forth slowly.

- **Brush below the gum line:** Don't stop with your teeth. Continue brushing even below the gum line to help remove bacteria.

- **Don't forget your tongue:** You also don't want to overlook your tongue. Brush the surface of it each time you brush your teeth. This will clean out germs and give you a fresh feel!

Review:
Our Recommendations for
Oral Care Products

These are the products that are most beneficial for patients on a regular basis:

Toothpaste:

Colgate® Total®

Why? Colgate® Total® is an overall excellent toothpaste choice, offering all kinds of benefits. It contains Triclosan, an antibacterial ingredient that works against plaque, tartar, gingivitis, and cavities. Plus, Colgate® Total® also strengthens enamel, helps gums, improves breath, and whitens teeth.

Desensitizing Toothpaste:

Sensodyne® Pronamel Toothpaste for Sensitive Teeth

Why? Gentle and effective, Sensodyne® Pronamel Toothpaste is an excellent toothpaste for patients with sensitive teeth. Chosen by *Dentistry Today* as one of the top 100 products of 2007 and clinically proven to relieve hypersensitivity in just two weeks, this toothpaste is designed to comfort and soothe nerves and harden softened enamel, in addition to offering all the benefits of regular toothpaste. That's why it remains the #1 dentist-recommended toothpaste of its kind.

Mouth Rinse:

The Natural Dentist® Healthy Gum Rinse

Why? We recommend The Natural Dentist® mouth rinse, both because it is effective and because it is made with all natural, safe ingredients. Created from herbal extracts, it helps treat even serious gum issues. Plus, it comes in two flavors: peppermint twist or orange zest.

Flossing Aid:

Waterpik® by Philips®

Why? Fun and effective, the Waterpik® is one of the best flossing tools on the market today. It's not only more enjoyable to use than traditional floss, but it's also more successful. According to one study, the Waterpik® is actually 93% more effective than string floss at reducing gingival bleeding.

Toothbrush:

Sonicare® Electric Toothbrush

Why? We have found that patients can actually be more effective with electric toothbrushes. Not only are they more enjoyable to use, but they also remove plaque in a way that manual toothbrushes can't.

Nutrition for a Healthy Mouth

Good nutrition plays an enormous role in the proper development and maintenance of healthy teeth and gums. Eating the right kinds of foods allows the teeth to grow strong and remain healthy, without improper bacteria or decay. While most patients know it's important to limit high-sugar drinks, a recent study has shown that they often don't realize how important fruits and vegetables can be.

Examine the foods you regularly consume, from drinks like soda and fruit juices to everyday snacks. If these foods are high in sugar, your risk of tooth decay is much higher. Try to limit daily juice intake to six ounces at most. Also, remember that the longer those sugars stay on the teeth, the more time they have to cause damage. Sugar-free gum after a sugary meal can help flush away the sugar from your teeth. Encourage a diet that's high in nutrition, filled with foods like vegetables and quality dairy products. Interestingly, a recent study shows something unexpected about the effects of dark chocolate on your oral health: by contrast to other sweets, dark chocolate actually cuts back on bacteria and plaque!

Foods that provide valuable nutrition and strengthen the teeth:

Vegetables, particularly dark, leafy ones like spinach, kale, broccoli, and bok choy
Dairy products like yogurt, milk, cheese, Peanut butter

Dark chocolate

Foods that can contribute to cavities:

Soda/pop
Candy and sweets
Starchy foods like bread, crackers, pretzels

Q: How important is calcium for my teeth?

A: Not only does calcium help build and maintain strong teeth, but it also develops healthy bones and helps prevent osteoporosis. Calcium keeps gums healthy, encourages teeth to grow and develop, and even protects against tooth decay. It can be found in foods like milk and other dairy products, as well as in dark and leafy vegetables such as spinach, broccoli, and bok choy.

CHAPTER 8

The Ultimate Solution

No matter what unique dental challenges a patient presents, there is a solution. Prospective patients do not need to feel embarrassed or ashamed; dental specialists have seen everything. There's no judgment or ridicule, but instead there are professionals who can guide patients on an easy path to a healthier, more functional, beautiful smile.

The way it works is simple. You come in, regardless of the condition of your teeth, and talk to an expert dentist who is well acquainted with oral problems, from chips to missing teeth to gum disease. It doesn't matter if you don't have all your teeth. Maybe some are broken, or maybe you've dealt with non-functional dentures. Whatever your background, age, gender, or other circumstances, you have hope through a treatment option proven to address all kinds of concerns.

The condition of your smile or who you are does not matter. There is a solution.

Oftentimes, the clients with severe dental problems are the same people who have high-profile positions that require professionals with pleasant demeanors and a nice smile. It's true of men and many women, too:

they're established, well-to-do patients with one big common denominator, and that is extreme dental fear or anxiety.

Because dental fear causes years or even decades of neglect, it's no surprise that patients who have this fear are then in need of comprehensive treatment. Of course, receiving that treatment seems to involve conquering the same fear that put them in the situation: that is where sedation comes in. With IV sedation, patients can rest peacefully in twilight while all the necessary treatments are performed quickly and effectively.

Whether the selected treatment involves implants, root canals, whitening, partial dentures, or veneers, through IV sedation, patients can walk out with an aesthetic, healthier smile in just a matter of hours. Some of the work may be of a temporary nature; in those cases where it is not final, the temporary restorations are very well made and look natural. It gives patients a way to function well, both socially and physically, which is the whole point of a comprehensive dental approach.

After one treatment, clients literally leave with a new smile! Any decay or gum disease is cleared up and treated. They can walk out of the office looking great, without disease, feeling confident and attractive—all in one brief afternoon.

Personal, Customized Plans

A customized plan is created for each individual patient, one that is going to be different for each person but that always guarantees the same powerful results.

Depending on the condition of a patient's smile, one dental visit could be all that's needed to fully restore a smile; in other more complex cases, additional visits may be needed. On average, more complex cases take about three to four visits. These are cases that require multiple root canals, implants, etc., because the patients' smiles are in such poor shape. It's important that the treatment plan be thorough and that it eradicate all decay and gum disease in order to transform an unhealthy mouth to a healthy mouth. Through a personal consultation with a specialist, a patient will get a better sense of what will be required.

The First Visit: What to Expect

Regardless of how many visits are required for your particular circumstances, you can be sure of this: you will leave your first visit with a functional, healthy, great-looking smile. You will be able to smile proudly and chew food normally after that first visit even if you require additional follow-up treatment. In some cases, the initial work will be temporary, but it will still be solid and attractive, giving you the confidence you wanted right away. Patients do not go home with missing or unstable teeth, and that is the wonderful part of the right plan.

When considering treatment, many people are concerned that they will have to walk around without teeth in the beginning. They understand that it takes some time to complete a major restoration and let the mouth fully heal. These are valid concerns; however, with the right specialists, you will never have to be without teeth. There are solutions specifically designed to prevent that from happening. That means you can rest assured that throughout the restoration process, you will look much more attractive than you did beforehand. You can go from an unhealthy state created by years of neglect and, in a few comfortable hours, have a totally different mouth and smile. You can have your confidence back in one afternoon. It's that simple.

Learning How to Smile Again

For patients who have spent years hiding their smiles, resisting that urge can be difficult. Not smiling has become a habit that has to be broken. People develop all kinds of weird ways to conceal their smiles when they are embarrassed about their teeth. Obviously, they don't look as good as they could when they depend on these habits, but psychologically they almost can't help it.

Those men who have been camouflaging their smiles with long moustaches, for example, work up the courage to shave them off. They may not do it immediately, as the decision can take time, but eventually those men will usually find the courage. They'll keep trimming their mustaches shorter and shorter until one day they're ready to let it go completely. It's like they're throwing away a security blanket: while it might not be easy to do, it's definitely worth it.

Similarly, those who have been hiding their smiles with their hands have to remind themselves there is nothing to hide anymore. After completing treatment, again in as little as one visit, patients emerge as new people, proud of their new smiles. They update their photos on their business websites; they look for ways to show off their teeth. Usually, they interact more successfully with clients, prospects, colleagues, and peers. A smiling person is always received more positively than one who doesn't smile or who displays peculiar habits trying to hide a smile. Often, patients will look at old photos and recognize the odd habits they used to resort to in order to camouflage their smiles, and they can't believe how far they've come.

The timing for realization that the days of an unattractive smile and the insecurities connected to it are over is different for everyone. Some leave the office and just can't stop smiling, catching their new facial expression in the windows, others take a little time to activate their "smiling" muscles. One of our patients described this feeling this way: "You know, when you learn a foreign language, it takes time and effort, but one day, all of a sudden, you realize that you understand and speak it." We want each restoration patient to be fluent in the language of smiling!

An Emotional Journey

Overcoming dental phobia is a significant emotional journey. After the makeover, clients emerge with a much more positive outlook on life and the future. Their confidence is restored. They have a better view of themselves, their family, their relationships, and their jobs. They often even look years younger. All of these emotional changes take place, opening a new world of possibilities for them, and there are also many accompanying changes, like losing weight, working out, and eating right to become healthier and look better. They start dating when they couldn't before. They experience improved love lives. They shave mustaches or color and cut their hair. Some get better jobs or start performing better in their current roles. A beautiful smile is a positive change that spurs other constructive changes.

"A smile is the light in your window that tells others that there is a caring, sharing person inside."
— Denis Waitley

CHAPTER 9

Success Stories

For countless patients, the long-postponed dental treatment has been an uplifting, exciting experience that has meant new confidence, new relationships, and even new lives. By receiving the dental care they so desperately needed, these people are living vibrant, active lives—no longer afraid to smile.

Tori's Story:

The Life-Changing Power of a Smile

A young, 30 year old Asian woman named Tori came to the dentist with significant tetracycline teeth staining—a problem that sometimes results from taking a certain antibiotic during childhood while adult teeth are still forming under the gums. Her entire set of teeth had unattractive permanent brown and gray stains—something that she was very self-conscious about.

Extremely shy and withdrawn, Tori was in the midst of medical school here in the United States. For her treatment, she received an entire mouthful of veneers. Because the procedure didn't require sedation, Tori talked to her dentist while she was placing the veneers. Tori said she hoped to do a residency in surgery, but her family wanted her to do it in radiology. She wasn't dating anyone. She didn't have many friends. She also mentioned that every time she went for a residency interview, she didn't get accepted, and she felt it was because she looked so unhappy and unhealthy because of her smile. That's actually what had prompted her to seek help in the first place: one of the doctors at the hospital where she'd last been interviewed had asked her about her teeth, "What's so weird with your smile? You don't look healthy." He didn't know she had tetracycline when she was a child, and that it had discolored her teeth, but the conversation impacted Tori.

After Tori received her veneers, her smile was completely different. She felt like a new woman. Soon after, she flew to California to attend some interviews for residency—and that's where her story gets really interesting.

Turns out, it wasn't only her smile that changed that day in the dental office; it was her entire person. Although Tori had the same face, she was not the same. Her entire demeanor was different. After she'd chosen dental surgery, she went to the California residency interviews and did very well. She landed the residency she'd wanted—in surgery. What's more, during the interview process, she'd met a man and later got engaged. Instead of the shy personality she'd previously had, she became happy and confident, with a beauty that radiated from her face. Just like that, her whole life had changed. While the only physical change was her smile—just some veneers in her mouth—the other changes that resulted were incredible. Even her expression was completely different. She became happy and confident. You could see it in her eyes.

The one change that made it all possible was her smile: that's what allowed her to be herself—and to land the surgical residency she wanted, as well as a fiancé.

While Tori's story may sound extreme, the truth is that these kinds of things happen all the time. Dental work is not just about a smile; it's about the person behind the smile. A new set of teeth can create an entire transformation of a person.

Natalie's Story

Natalie was an investment banker who hadn't had major dental treatment for about a year. When she came in for a routine cleaning, she needed sedation even for that. Afterwards, her dentist asked about her new smile, and she quickly explained, "Oh, I just love it." She said it didn't take her long to get used to smiling again. In fact, she said she smiled right away when she walked out of the office and that the treatment changed her life immediately.

Like Natalie, a lot of patients start smiling the day they receive treatment, but some other people are not like that. For some patients, it takes a good amount of time for them to learn how to smile again. It's like physical therapy: when a person has to learn to walk again after a traumatic event, it may take some get-

ting used to. The brain still remembers, but putting that memory into practice takes time, just like learning how to walk again.

Kevin's Story:

A Second Chance at Life and Love

Kevin was a 58 year old man and father of two—a child who was 29 and a child who was six. He'd had his younger son through his second marriage, which was to a much younger woman; he was in his early fifties when that son was born.

When Kevin came to the dentist, his smile was in real trouble. He was missing teeth, his gums were unhealthy, and several teeth were severely decayed. Yet at the same time, he was dressed very nicely, enjoyed a stable and high-powered job, and had so much going for him. As is often the case with men in his situation who are ashamed of their teeth, Kevin wore a very long mustache to help cover his smile. It wasn't like he was unattractive; he just lacked confidence in that one area, and so he wanted to try and hide his face.

Kevin fit the classic profile of having dental phobia: he'd had a bad dental experience as a kid, and because of that past, he'd avoided the dentist for years, creating a host of dental problems. For most of his life, he didn't smile, but at the same time, he wanted to be able to enjoy life. Plus, on top of that, he had a young child and a younger wife, so he wanted to feel younger.

As Kevin's dental treatment progressed, so did his transformation. As his smile improved, so did his habits: he started working out, he colored his hair, he started going out with his kids, he took his family to Disneyland. Prompted by his dental treatment, Kevin changed tremendously: he looked much younger, and he found himself enjoying life to the fullest, smiling proudly. Today, he says his only regret is that he didn't seek help sooner.

Damon's Story:

Even Scaredy Cats Want New Smiles

Although all patients are different, their stories are often very similar. Most people need lots of work, many have experienced negative dental work as children, many are truly terrified of seeing a dentist or having work done in their mouths. There are also those patients who have severe dental phobias and don't know how to conquer them. That's where IV sedation plays such a key role. It's truly the gold standard of dentistry and the tool that helps patients wake up with new smiles.

Damon was a patient who came in with a severe dental phobia. A successful small business owner in New York, he was absolutely terrified of stepping into a dental office, not to mention undergoing treatment. It took a lot of courage for him to even seek help. The good news is, though, that by the time his treatments were completed, not only did his smile change, his life did as well. His eyes changed. His skin changed. His attitude changed. Today, he looks healthier, younger, and more energetic. As is the case for so many patients, all of these positive improvements came just from treating his smile.

"When you see that many people with a smile on their face, then you must be doing something right."

— Greg Norman

Patient Testimonials

"What I have loved about coming to Smile in the City is that there has been no pain, no judgment, and no lectures. I wasn't yelled at about the past. I had significant dental problems but waiting and waiting for years didn't make it go away! The positive results I received from Smile in the City was that it motivated me to take care of the rest of me and I went on a diet. So between my smile and my weight - people who I take the train with and buy my coffee from - people who I didn't think pay attention to me have told me out of the blue that I look great. It's happened many times. (It never happened before!). Thank You to the wonderful team at Smile in the City."
— Jim B.

"All my past visits to any dentist have been filled with anxiety, dread, and overall fear. First off, the entire staff at Smile in the City was confident and pleasant and gave me a most comfortable feeling. Dr. Zelig and Dr.

Schmidt were truly professional and compassionate. Their procedures were perfectly orchestrated and the most relaxing and totally pain free process I had ever experienced. I don't know why I didn't look sooner. They can expect a life-time patient. Thank you all."
— Oliver S.

"Visits to the dentist's office were a source of terrifying fear for me in the past. I have now put that fear behind me. Dr. Zelig and associates are professionals through & through. I had the first truly painless dental work done in my life. I can proudly say, "I have the best dentist"! I would highly recommend their services to everyone. I have finally found a dentist who understands the fear I had and is true to his word when he says he will not hurt you."

— Ann Marie A.

"Dr. Z. is one of a kind!! & his office is made up of some of the most caring & gentle people I have come to know whilst being in NYC. I am from South Africa, but living in NYC as a model. Until meeting him and his colleagues, I had always avoided going to the dentist, as I HAD a terrible fear, which began as a child. I never faced it, until on a flight back to the states after a job, I felt my tooth start to ache so badly, I knew I

had to see one, so when I got back I googled Dentist that do IV sedation in NYC, as I knew this would be the only way I would have a procedure. After reading many testimonials, viewing the website & seeing pictures of his office, I could tell it offered a calming ambience & didn't come across as a cold dentistry office. I called to make an appointment. On the day of it everyone was so kind & could tell I was so nervous so spoke to me in such a way that it lifted my spirits and made me relax. It turned out I needed a root canal. Dr. Z. kept his promise to me and never began anything till I was completely relaxed, he gave me beautiful calming music to listen to & then the IV sedation. I never felt a thing! :) I was amazed, and NO swelling the next day!!! He is the BEST!! :)"
— *Lisa M.*

When I first met with Dr. Reiner and told him about my mouse phobia, he immediately put me at ease. He listened carefully and emphatically and assured me that in the span of just a few months I would be able to have a mouse crawl on me while remaining calm. Of course, I looked at him like he was crazy and doubted that the treatment would ever be successful. But I was also sick of living in fear and so I decided to take a leap of faith and put my trust in Dr. Reiner. This turned out to be a great decision.

Over the course of the treatment, Dr. Reiner slowly and gradually helped to desensitize me to mice. He had me start off by viewing images of mice before exposing me to live mice. Meanwhile, he taught me simple relaxation techniques that helped me to tolerate my anxiety during this process. He also hooked me up to biofeedback equipment to show me that I could control my body's anxiety response – this discovery was very empowering. Throughout all of this, Dr. Reiner was extraordinarily patient with me and helped me to feel like I was in charge of the process at all times. By the time I graduated from treatment (just a few months after I had begun treatment), I was able to have a mouse run across my foot (my greatest fear prior to embarking on treatment!) while calmly engaging in conversation. I never in a million years thought that I would be able to achieve this, considering I couldn't even be in the same room as a mouse when I started treatment.

My husband could not believe it either and feels very proud of the progress that I've achieved. I feel incredible gratitude towards Dr. Reiner for helping me to shed this irksome phobia that has interfered with my life for too long. I know that I could never have made these gains without his patience, expert guidance, and encouragement.

I would encourage anyone who is dealing with a phobia to not hesitate to seek help from Dr. Reiner -- he is simply the best at what he does. Don't get me wrong, the process can feel difficult at times and progress may not always be purely linear. However, if you invest in the treatment and allow Dr. Reiner to guide you than I have no doubt that you will be as successful as I have been in improving the quality of your life.
— Linda M.

EPILOGUE

Dr. Robert H. Reiner

When I was first approached by Doctors Zelig and Schmidt in the spring of 2011 to contribute to their book on dental phobias I was intrigued by the opportunity to shed some light on our common ground. After all, as a psychologist, I have been working closely with dentists for decades, often treating their referred patients for a variety of issues ranging from stress related muscular/myofacial problems like bruxism (teeth grinding), temporomandibular joint syndrome (TMJ; essentially a headache in the jaw), anxiety/depression, public speaking anxiety, all the way to dental phobia. From the perspective of a psychologist and pain specialist, both the jaw and the mouth receive inordinate amounts of attention.

What other joint in the human body moves in three directions, up and down, back and forward, and side to side? We use the mouth for such a wide range of things; just to name a few, speaking, chewing, breathing, kissing, smiling, tasting, drinking, spitting, storing, yawning, snoring, biting, sucking, licking and vomiting. The intimacy associated with the functions of the mouth coupled with the presence of complex, high frequency/highly sensitive nerve endings make it understandable that so many people are afraid to visit conventional dentists. For this reason, patients with dental phobias should only consult experienced dentists with advanced specialized training.

Although I have been practicing clinical psychology on Manhattan's upper east side for more than thirty years, I continue to get a unique thrill from observing the outcome of merging technologies. Psychology and dentistry have both been recent recipients of dramatic technological advances. As the founder and executive director of Behavioral Associates, one of New York's oldest and largest outpatient CBT* oriented psychotherapy institutes, my experience reveals that each new project involving overlapping technologies has lead to results that have been exciting and often unpredictable. At this point in my career, with a professional staff of approximately 20 psychiatrists, psychologists, and psychiatric social workers, time constraints limit me to personally treating only a dozen or so individual psychotherapy patients per week. Besides teaching and supervising my staff, I do all the initial intakes and determine which patients and therapists I believe will match up best. Meeting four or five new patients every day, after all these years, has provided a unique opportunity to understand just how much each stage of life has predictable priorities. These are important considerations in making what are potentially life changing decisions for the 400 patients seen by our staff, on a weekly basis.

After reading their manuscript, the major reason I requested deeper involvement was the realization that the technological advances that served as backbones of treatment methodology for our two professions has so much in common. It turns out that the anchors for the "cure points" of dentistry (IV sedation) and psychology (RSA assisted diaphragmatic breathing) serve almost identical purposes. As the attentive reader now understands, IV sedation and biofeedback assisted abdominal breathing procedures both provide very pleasurable, anxiety free experiences. It is this very pairing of pleasure with the anxiety producing experience, that serves to re-direct and ultimately restructure feelings of fear and inhibition in the direction of behavioral freedom and regained sense of control.

About the Doctors

Joseph Zelig, D.D.S.
Diplomate, American Board of Periodontology

Dr. Zelig is a board certified periodontist practicing at Smile in the City Dental Group in New York City, NY. He is skilled in all phases of laser periodontal treatment including surgical and non-surgical pocket reduction, regeneration and grafting, cosmetic root coverage procedures, and aesthetic crown lengthening. He is also an expert in all aspects of surgical dental implant placement including advanced bone grafting/ridge augmentation, socket preservation and sinus grafting. In addition, Dr. Zelig holds a permit in intravenous conscious sedation from the New York State Board of Dentistry and is fully trained and qualified to perform intravenous or IV sedation.

Dr. Zelig earned a doctorate of dental surgery degree from New York University College of Dentistry. He then completed an additional three years of course and clinical work specializing in Periodontics through New York University College of Dentistry Advanced Education. Through his training, Dr. Zelig learned the art and science of periodontics and implantology from some of the best periodontists in the country.

Dr. Zelig holds many active memberships in dental and periodontal professional organizations such as American Board of Periodontology, American Academy of Periodontology, American Society for Dental Anesthesiology, Northeastern Society of Periodontists, and others.

In addition, Dr. Zelig serves as president of the New York Center for Advanced Dental Education. In this role, he is actively involved in sharing his expertise by teaching periodontics and implant dentistry to other dentists and specialists. Dr. Zelig spends a great deal of his time lecturing, educating and training others in the field. Dr. Zelig also serves on the Advisory Committee of the Dental Implant Training Center in New Jersey.

Dr. Zelig has also given presentations at the Greater New York Dental Convention, the Northeastern Society of Periodontists and the Metropolitan Periodontal Symposium.

 Dr. Zelig's decision to become a dentist was an emotional one. He himself went through a very difficult time as a young adult dealing with severe dental phobia. Through the care of a skilled dental sedation specialist, Dr. Zelig managed to free himself from the burden of anxiety and to undergo extensive dental work. Now, Dr. Zelig devotes his career to helping those who suffer from dental anxiety by treating his patients with care and understanding.

Dr. Zelig possesses a warm and friendly "chair-side" manner and it is his innate warmth, patience, and sincerity that make the difference in his care.

Nargiz Schmidt, D.D.S.

Dr. Nargiz Schmidt is a prosthodontist practicing at Smile in the City Dental Group in New York City, NY. As a prosthodontist, she is a dental specialist skilled in reconstructive, aesthetic, and implant dentistry.

Dr. Schmidt received a doctoral degree from State University of New York at Stony Brook School of Dental Medicine with numerous awards for academic and clinical achievements in pharmacology, clinical dentistry, and biochemistry. After spending two years in private practice as a general dentist, Dr. Schmidt went back to school to become a specialist in cosmetic and reconstructive dentistry.

She was accepted into the New York University College of Dentistry Advanced Education program in prosthodontics. She learned the art and science of prosthodontics and aesthetic dentistry from some of the best specialists in the country. Following the completion of this three-year full-time program, Dr. Schmidt received certification as a prosthodontist.

With vast knowledge in complex dental restorations and rehabilitation, Dr. Schmidt often serves as a consultant to general dentists and other dental specialists and receives referrals from them.

Dr. Schmidt is devoted to her profession and never stops learning innovative techniques and materials available in today's dentistry. She is certified in Invisalign, a system that uses clear, removable aligners to gradually move teeth, as well as Lumineers, noninvasive porcelain laminate veneers. Using this advanced dental technology, she can transform your smile painlessly without removal of tooth structure.

Dentistry is a combination of science, engineering, craftsmanship, art, and psychology. Dr. Schmidt believes it's like no other profession, and she loves it because it is what allows her to strive for greatness.

As a prosthodontist, Dr. Schmidt is sensitively attuned to the aesthetic and functional concerns of her patients. She combines her scientific background with an artistic eye to bring the highest quality of personalized care to each of her patients. Dr. Nargiz Schmidt is a caring, gentle, and understanding professional. She will listen to your concerns and will address each and every of them in her treatments.

Robert H. Reiner, Ph.D.

Dr. Reiner is internationally recognized as a leading authority on treating phobias and anxiety disorders. He is the founder and executive director of Behavioral Associates, a clinical and consulting psychological institute located on Manhattan's Upper East Side. Behavioral Associates, staffed by 21 psychiatrists, psychologists, and psychiatric social workers, provides outpatient health psychology care to approximately 400 patients per week.

Dr. Reiner has been a member of the Department of Psychiatry of New York University Medical Center for over 30 years and has served as a psychological consultant for a variety of corporations. He received his Ph.D. in clinical psychology at the University of Alabama, his B.A. from the University of Pennsylvania and served his clinical internship at Bellevue Hospital.

Dr. Reiner was a guest lecturer at the International Virtual Reality Conference in Laval, France in 2001, presenting his landmark paper pioneering the utilization of biofeedback as an adjunct to virtual reality treatment(s). He was recently asked again to present his work at his old alma mater, The University of Pennsylvania Psychology Dept., a lecture series he presented for the first time last April. He has been invited back to repeat it for the spring of 2012. Interested readers are referred to www.behavioralassociates.com

i.   Berggren, U., and G. Meynert. "Dental fear and avoidance: causes, symptoms, and consequences." J Am Dent Assoc. 1984
Aug;109(2):247-51.

ii.   Lahti, S., and A. Luoto. "Significant relationship between parental and child dental fear." Evid Based Dent. 2010;11(3):77.

iii.   Rosted, P., M. Bundgaard, S. Gordon, and A.M. Pedersen.
"Acupuncture in the management of anxiety related to dental treatment: a
case series." Acupunct Med. 2010 Mar;28(1):3-5.

iv.   Lu, D.P., G.P. Lu, and J.F. Reed 3rd. "Acupuncture/acupressure
to treat gagging dental patients: a clinical study of anti-gagging effects." Gen
Dent. 2000 Jul-Aug;48(4):446-52.

v.   Manzoni, Mauro, Francesco Pagnini, Gianluca Castelnuovo,
and Enrico Molinari. "Relaxation training for anxiety: a ten-year systematic
review with meta-analysis." BMC Psychiatry. 2008; 8: 41. Published online
2008 June 2. Doi: 10.1186/1471-244X-8-41.

vi.   Forgione, A.G. "Hypnosis in the treatment of dental fear and
phobia." Dent Clin North Am. 1988 Oct;32(4):745-61.

vii.   De Jongh, A., and D.L. Broers. "Risks of dental fear reduction
treatments." Ned Tijdschr Tandheelkd. 2009 Jun;116(6):324-9.

viii.   Armfield, Jason M., Judy F. Stewart, and A. John Spencer. "The
vicious cycle of dental fear: exploring the interplay between oral health,
service utilization and dental fear." BMC Oral Health. 2007; 7: 1. Published
online 2007 January 14. Doi: 10.1186/1472-6831-7-1.

ix.   Schwilden, H., and J. Schuttler. "200 years of nitrous oxide
(laughing gas)—and the end of an era?" Anasthesiol Intensivmed Not-
fallmed Schmerzther. 2001 Oct;36(10):640.

x.   Sokolowski, C.J., J.A. Jr Giovannitti, and S.G. Boynes. "Needle
phobia: etiology, adverse consequences, and patient management." Dental
Clin North Am. 2010 Oct;54(4):731-44.

xi.   Fischman, S. L. (1997). "The history of oral hygiene products:
how far have we come in 6000 years?". Periodontology 2000, 15: 7–14. doi:
10.1111/j.1600-0757.1997.tb00099.x

xii.   Jefferson, Eugenia. "Chewing gum might reduce dental caries."
Journal of Dental Hygiene, 82.5 (Fall 2008).

xiii.   American Dental Association. "Whitening Toothpastes." J Am
Dent Assoc, Vol 132, No 8, 1146-1147.

xiv.   Joiner, A. "Whitening toothpastes: A review of the literature." J
Dent. 2010 May 24. PMID: 20562012.

xv.   Carmona, Richard H., MD, MPH, FACS. "Statement on Water

Fluoridation." National Institute of Dental and Craniofacial Research, July 2004. http://www.nidcr.nih.gov/OralHealth/Topics/Fluoride/Statement-WaterFluoridation.htm

xvi.   The Office of the Surgeon General. The Benefits of Fluoride. U.S. Department of Health and Human Services, May 2000. http://www.cdc.gov/fluoridation/fact_sheets/benefits.htm

xvii.   American Dental Association. "Cleaning Your Teeth & Gums." http://www.ada.org/2624.aspx

xviii.   "How Do I Choose and Use a Toothbrush?" Oral Health Resources, Hygiene. Academy of General Dentistry. 29 March 2007. http://www.agd.org/support/articles/?ArtID=1212

xix.   Warren, Paul R., L.D.S., Tonya Smith Ray, RDH, MA, Maryann Cugini, RDH, MHP, and Bernard V. Chater, PhD. "A practice-based study of a power toothbrush: assessment of effectiveness and acceptance." The Journal of the American Dental Association, Volume 131, No 3, 389-394. 2000.

xx.   American Dental Association. "Cleaning Your Teeth & Gums." http://www.ada.org/2624.aspx

xxi.   Barnes, C.M., C.M. Russell, R.A. Reinhardt, J.B. Payne, and D.M. Lyle. "Waterpik® Water Flossers: More Effective Than String Floss for Reducing Gingivitis." Journal of Clinical Dentistry, 2005: 16(3):71-77.

xxii.   "Bad Breath (Halitosis)." American Dental Association. http://www.ada.org/2941.aspx?currentTab=1

xxiii.   "Cleaning Your Teeth & Gums." American Dental Association. http://www.ada.org/3072.aspx?currentTab=1

xxiv.   Yaskell, Tina, Anne D. Haffajee, and Sigmund S. Socransky. "Antimicrobial effectiveness of an herbal mouthrinse against predominant oral bacteria species in vitro." Journal of Dental Hygiene, 81.4-5 (Fall 2007).

xxv.   Mouthrinses. American Dental Association. http://www.ada.org/1319.aspx

xxvi.   Gallagher, Andrew, Joseph Sowinski, James Bowman, Kathy Barrett, Shirley Lowe, Kartik Patel, Mary Lynn Bosma, and Jonathan E. Creeth. "The effect of brushing time and dentifrice on dental plaque removal in vivo." Journal of Dental Hygiene, 83.3 (Summer 2009): p111(6).

xxvii.   GSK data on file, support study #111-062-05.

xxviii.   GSK data on file, support study #111-062-05.

xxix.   Barnes, C.M., C.M. Russell, R.A. Reinhardt, J.B. Payne, and D.M. Lyle. "Waterpik® Water Flossers: More Effective Than String Floss for Reducing Gingivitis." Journal of Clinical Dentistry, 2005: 16(3):71-77.

xxx.   Wiener, R. Constance, Richard J. Crout, and Michael A. Wiener. "Toothpaste use by children, oral hygiene, and nutritional education:
an assessment of parental performance." Journal of Dental Hygiene, 83.3
(Summer 2009): p141(5).

xxxi.   "Inhibitory effects of cacao bean husk extract on plaque formation in vitro and in vivo." European Journal of Oral Sciences. 2004 Vol. 112,
Issue 3, 249.

xxxii.   Hurst, P.S., L.H. Lacey, and A.H. Crisp. "Teeth, vomiting and
diet: a study of the dental characteristics of seventeen anorexia nervosa
patients." Postgrad Med J. 1977 Jun;53(630):298-305.

xxxiii.   Lazarchik, D.A., and K.B. Frazier. "Dental erosion and acid
reflux disease: an overview." Gen Dent. 2009 Mar-April;57(2):151-6; quiz
157-8.

xxxiv.   Gonzalez-Cabezas, C. "The chemistry of caries: remineralization
and demineralization events with direct clinical relevance." Dent Clin North
Am. 2010 Jul;54(3):469-78.

xxxv.   Cochrane, N.J., F. Cai, N.L. Huq, M.F. Burrow, and E.C. Reyn-
olds. "New Approaches to Enhanced Remineralization of Tooth Enamel." J
Dent Res. 2010 Aug 25.

xxxvi.   Hemmings, Ken, Brigitte Griffiths, John Hobkirk, and Crispian
Scully. "Improving occlusion and orofacial aesthetics: tooth repair and
replacement." BMJ. 2000 August 12; 321(7258): 438-441.

xxxvii.   Meyer, A. Jr, L.C. Cardoso, E. Araujo, and L.N. Baratieri. "Ceramic inlays and onlays: clinical procedures for predictable results."
xxxviii. Roberts, H.W., and D.G. Charlton. "The release of mercury from
amalgam restorations and its health benefits: a review." Oper Dent. 2009
Sep-Oct;34(5):605-14.

xxxix.   Review and Analysis of the Literature on the Potential Health
Effects of Dental Amalgams. 2004 December 9. http://www.lsro.org/amal-
gam/frames_amalgam_home.html

xl.   Mozes, Alan. "Fillings, Sealants May Leach BPA into Kids'
Mouths." HealthDay, U.S. Department of Health & Human Services. 7
September 2010.

xli.   Tysowsky, G.W. "The science behind lithium disilicate: a metal-
free alternative." Dent Today. 2009 Mar;28(3):112-3.

xlii.   Wong, M., and W.R. Lytle. "A comparison of anxiety levels associated with root canal therapy and oral surgery treatment." J Endod. 1991
Sep;17(9):461-5.

xliii.   Seguar-Egea, J.J., R. Cisneros-Cabello, J.M. Llamas-Carreras, E. Velasco-Ortega. "Pain associated with root canal treatment." Int Endod J. 2009 Jul;42(7):614-20. Epub 2009 May 8.

xliv.   Balto, K. "How common is tooth pain after root canal treatment?" Evid Based Dent. 2010;11(4):114.

xlv.   Zhang, F., F. Wang, and Y.L. Wang. "Investigation of dental anxiety on root canal treatment." Dept of Stomatology, China-Japan Friendship Hospital, Beijing 100029, China.

xlvi.   Newton, J.T. "Music may reduce anxiety during invasive procedures in adolescents and adults." J Clin Nurs. 2008 Oct;17(19):2654-60.

xlvii.   Dugas, N.N., H.P. Lawrence, P. Teplitsky, S. Friedman. "Quality of life and satisfaction outcomes of endodontic treatment." J Endod. 2002 Dec;28(12):819-27.

xlviii.   Barnes, J.J., S. Patel, and F. Mannocci. "Why do general dental practitioners refer to a specific specialist endodontist in practice?" Int Endod J. 2011 Jan;44(1):21-32. Doi: 10.1111/j. 1365-2591.2010.01791.x. Epub 2010 Aug 31.

xlix.   Ryan, W., and A. O'Connel. "The attitudes of undergraduate dental students to the use of the rubber dam." J Ir Dental Assoc. 2007 Summer;53(2):87-91.

l.   Slawinski, D., and S. Wilson. "Rubber dam use: a survey of pediatric dentistry training programs and private practitioners." Pediatr Dent. 2010 Jan-Feb;32(1):64-8.

li.   "Gum Disease Found to Be Significant Public Health Concern." American Academy of Periodontology. 21 September 2010.

lii.   "Dispelling Myths about Gum Disease: The Truth behind Healthy Teeth and Gums." American Academy of Periodontology. 18 February 2010. http://www.perio.org/consumer/gum-disease-myths.htm

liii.   Michalowicz, Dr. Bryan S., Scott R. Diehl, John C. Gunsolley, Brandon S. Sparks, Carol N. Brooks, Thomas E. Koertge, Joseph V. Califano, John A. Burmeister, and Harvey A. Schenkein. "Evidence of a Substantial Genetic Basis for Risk of Adult Periodontitis." Journal of Periodontology. November 2000, Vol. 71, No. 11, Pages 1699-1707.

liv.   Asikainen, S., C. Chen, S. Alalussua, and J. Slots. "Can one acquire periodontal bacteria and periodontitis from a family member?". Journal of the American Dental Association, September 1997, Vol 128, Issue 9, 1263-1271.

lv.   Albandar, Dr. J.M., J. A. Brunelle, and A. Kingman. "Destructive Periodontal Disease in Adults 30 Years of Age and Older in the United

States, 1988-1994." Journal of Periodontology. January 1999, Vol. 70, No. 1, Pages 13-29.

lvi.   Kibayaski, Miyuki, Muneo Tanaka, Nobuko Nishida, Nasae Kuboniwa, Kosuke Kataoka, Hideki Nagata, Kunio Nakayama, Kanehisa Morimoto, and Satoshi Shizukuishi. "Longitudinal Study of the Association between Smoking as a Periodontitis Risk and Salivary Biomarkers Related to Periodontitis." Journal of Periodontology. May 2007, Vol. 78, No. 5, Pages 859-867.

lvii.   Getulio da R. Nogueria-Filho, Bruno Trevisan Rosa, Joao B. Cesar-Neto, Roberto S. Tunes, and Urbino da R. Tunes. "Low- and High-Yield Cigarette Smoke Inhalation Potentiates Bone Loss During Ligature-Induced Periodontitis." Gum Disease. April 2007, Vol. 78, No. 4, Pages 730-735.

lviii.   Tomar, Dr. Scott L., and Samira Asma. "Smoking-Attributable Periodontitis in the United States: Findings from NHANES III." Journal of Periodontology. May 2000, Vol. 71, No. 5, Pages 743-751.

lix.   Ayangco, Lilibeth, and Dr. Philip J. Sheridan. "Minocycline-Induced Staining of Torus Palatinus and Alveolar Bone." Journal of Periodontology. May 2003, Vol. 74, No. 5, Pages 669-671.

lx.   Ilgenli, Tunc, Dr. Gul Atilla, and Haluk Baylas. "Effectiveness of Periodontal Therapy in Patients with Drug-Induced Gingival Overgrowth. Long-Term Results." Journal of Periodontology. September 1999, Vol. 70, No. 9, Pages 967-972.

lxi.   Cutler, Dr. Christopher W., Robert L. Machen, Ravi Jotwani, and Anthony M. Iacopino. "Heightened Gingival Inflammation and Attachment Loss in Type 2 Diabetics with Hyperlipidemia." Journal of Periodontology. November 1999, Vol. 70, No. 11, Pages 1313-1321.

lxii.   Genco, R.J., S.G. Grossi, A. Ho, F. Nishimura, and Y. Murayama. "A proposed model linking inflammation to obesity, diabetes, and periodontal infections." Journal of Periodontology. 2005 Nov;76(11 Suppl):2075-84.

lxiii.   Nishida, Mieko, Sara G. Grossi, Robert G. Dunford, Alex W. Ho, Maurizio Trevisan, and Robert J. Genco. "Dietary Vitamin C and the Risk for Periodontal Disease." Journal of Periodontology. August 2000, Vol. 71, No. 8, Pages 1215-1223.

lxiv.   Peruzzo, Daiane C., Bruno B. Benatti, Glaucia M.B. Ambrosano, Getulio R. Nogueira-Filho, Enilson A. Sallum, Marcio Z. Casati, and Francisco H. Nociti Jr. "A Systematic Review of Stress and Psychological Factors as Possible Risk Factors for Periodontal Disease." Journal of Periodontology. August 2007, Vol. 78, No. 8, Pages 1491-1504.

lxv.   Hugo, Fernando N., Juliana B. Hilgert, Mary C. Bozzetti, Denise R. Bandeira, Tonantzin R. Goncalves, Josiane Pawlowski, and Maria da Luz R. de Sousa. "Chronic Stress, Depression, and Cortisol Levels as Risk Indicators of Elevated Plaque and Gingivitis Levels in Individuals Aged 50 Years and Older." Journal of Periodontology. June 2006, Vol. 77, No. 6, Pages 1008-1014.

lxvi.   Mullally, Brian H., Wilson A. Coulter, Julia D. Hutchinson, and Heather A. Clarke. "Current Oral Contraceptive Status and Periodontitis in Young Adults." Journal of Periodontology. June 2007, Vol. 78, No. 6, Pages 1031-1036.

lxvii.   Mustapha, Indra Z., Sarah Debrey, Michael Oladubu, and Richard Ugarte. "Makers of Systemic Bacterial Exposure in Periodontal Disease and Cardiovascular Disease Risk: A Systematic Review and Meta-Analysis." Journal of Periodontology. December 2007, Vol. 78, No. 12, Pages 2289-2302.

lxviii.   Michaud, Dr. Dominque S ScD, Yan Liu MS, Mara Meyer ScM, Prof. Edward Giovannucci ScD, and Prof. Kaumudi Joshipura ScD. "Periodontal disease, tooth loss, and cancer risk in male health professionals: a prospective cohort study." The Lancet Oncology. Volume 9, Issue 6, Pages 550-558, June 2008.

lxix.   Shimazaki, Yoshihiro, Yuko Egami, Takeshi Matsubara, George Koike, Sumio Akifusa, Sumie Jingu, and Yoshihisa Yamashita. "Relationship between Obesity and Physical Fitness and Periodontitis." Journal of Periodontology. 2010, Vol. 81, No. 8, Pages 1124-1131.

lxx.   Nishida, Mieko, Sara G. Grossi, Robert G. Dunford, Alex W. Ho, Maurizio Trevisan, and Robert J. Genco. "Calcium and the Risk for Periodontal Disease." Journal of Periodontology. July 2000, Vol. 71, No. 7, Pages 1057-1066.

lxxi.   Boj, Juan/Galofre, Neus/Espana, Antoi/Espasa, Enric. "Pain Perception in Pediatric Patients Undergoing Laser Treatments." Journal of Oral Laser Applications. Year 2005, Volume 5, Issue 2, Pages 85-89.

lxxii.   Zlataric, D.K., A. Celebic, and M. Valentic-Peruzovic. "The effect of removable partial dentures on periodontal health of abutment and non-abutment teeth." J Periodontol. 2002 Feb;73(2):137-44.

lxxiii.   Henry, P.J. "Tooth loss and implant replacement." Aust Dent J. 2000 Sep;45(3): 150-72.

lxxiv.   Schropp, L., and F. Isidor. "Timing of implant placement relative to tooth extraction." J Oral Rehabil. 2008 Jan;35 Suppl 1:33-43.

lxxv.   Leary, J.C., and M. Hirayama. "Extraction, immediate-load implants, impressions and final restorations in two patient visits." J Am Dent Assoc. 2003 Jun;134(6):715-20.

lxxvi.   Cannizzaro, G., M. Leone, U. Consolo, V. Ferri, and M. Esposito. "Immediate functional loading of implants placed with flapless surgery versus conventional implants in partially edentulous patients: a 3-year randomized controlled clinical trial." Int J Oral Maxillofac Implants. 2008 Sep-Oct;23(5):867-75.

lxxvii.   Kacer, C.M., J.D. Dyer, and R.A. Kraut. "Immediate loading of dental implants in the anterior and posterior mandible: a retrospective study of 120 cases." J Oral Maxillofac Surg. 2010 Nov;68(11):2861-7.

lxxviii.   Esposito, M., M.G. Grusovin, I.P. Polyzos, P. Felice, and H.V. Worthington. "Timing of implant placement after tooth extraction: immediate, immediate-delayed or delayed implants?" Eur J Oral Implantol. 2010 Autumn;3(3): 189-205.

lxxix.   Bilhan, H., E. Mumcu, and S. Arat. "The role of timing of loading on later marginal bone loss around dental implants: a retrospective clinical study." J Oral Implantol. 2010;36(5):363-76. Epub 2010 June 14.

lxxx.   Esfandiari, S., J.P. Lund, J.R. Penrod, A. Savard, J.M. Thomason, and J.S. Feine. "Implant overdentures for edentulous elders: study of patient preference." Gerodontology. 2009 Mar;26(1):4-20. Epub 2008 May 20.

lxxxi.   Balaguer, J., B. Garcia, M.A. Penarrocha, and M. Penarrocha. "Satisfaction of patients fitted with implant-retained overdentures." Med Oral Patol Oral Cir Bucal. 2010 Aug 15.

lxxxii.   Van der Bilt, A., M. Burgers, FMC van Kampen, M.S. Cune. "Mandibular implant-supported overdentures and oral function." Clin. Oral Impl. Res. 21, 2010; 1209-1213.
doi: 10.1111/j.1600-0501.2010.01915.x.

lxxxiii.   Depprich, Rita, Holger Zipprich, Michelle Ommerborn, Christian Naujoks, Hans-Peter Wiesmann, Sirichai Kiattavorncharoen, Hans-Christoph Lauer, Ulrich Meyer, Norbert R. Kubler, and Jorg Handschel. "Osseointegration of zirconia implants compared with titanium: an in vivo study." Head Face Med. 2008; 4:30. Published online 2008 December 11. Doi 10.1186/1746-160X-4-30.

lxxxiv.   Vagkopoulou, T., S.O. Koutayas, P. Koidis, and J.R. Strub. "Zirconia in dentistry: Part 1. Discovering the nature of an upcoming bioceramic." Eur J Esthet Dent. 2009 Summer;4(2):130-51.